NEW LIFE FOR MILLIONS:

Rehabilitation for America's Disabled

NEW LIFE FOR MILLIONS:

Rehabilitation for America's Disabled

by

RUSSELL J. N. DEAN

HASTINGS HOUSE, PUBLISHERS

NEW YORK

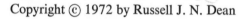

Copyright © 1972 by Russell J. N. Dean

Published simultaneously in Canada by
Saunders of Toronto, Ltd., Don Mills, Ontario

Library of Congress Catalog Card Number; 72-2000

Library of Congress Cataloging in Publication Data
Dean, Russell J   N   Date
  New life for millions: rehabilitation for America's disabled
  1. Rehabilitation—United States—History.
I. Title.
HD7256.U5D4   362.4'0973   72-2000
ISBN 0-8038-5024-7

Printed in the United States of America

CONTENTS

——◄••••►——

PHOTOGRAPHS

———•••———

FOREWORD

———◆◆◆►———

THIS IS A VIVID recounting of both the known and unknown
aspects of one of the most dynamic and dramatic movements
of modern times, which has sent and still sends action waves
to countries and continents far from American shores.

This book tells the story of the unusual people who
gave us today's often-miraculous programs for rescuing seriously disabled people from oblivion. The "rehabilitation
movement" in this country has been, for the most part, a
quiet movement. Now, rehabilitation's three score and ten
years in America come alive in this moving résumé of the
lives and times of those remarkable rehabilitation people.

As a beneficiary myself of the military and veterans'
rehabilitation programs during World War II, and as an active volunteer the past quarter century, I now have a clearer,
brighter picture of events of which I was a part, thanks to
the style, thrust and research of this volume.

Centered around the chief actors in the 20th Century
drama of rehabilitation, the author has chosen his giants
well in naming Milbank, Kratz, Kessler, Krusen, Rusk and
Switzer to his 70-year rehabilitation "Hall of Fame." Few

will quarrel with his choice of giants, all of whom he knew personally, for he has given almost all the actors their time on stage as he moves from military to civilian services, from public to private programs, medicine to paramedical, facilities to research, dreams to fulfillment.

A knowledgeable and skillful bureaucrat for many years, lobbyist and writer, Dean has brought to *New Life for Millions* his own rich background of personal association with most of the major organizations recorded.

His thoughtful Epilogue must not be lost to those of us who remain on stage. The work is not yet done. Please God, it will be done in our own time. If not, this volume will help speed that day. Those who read it with nostalgia will be encouraged to persevere. Those who come on later will take what we have wrought and renew and improve upon it in the years ahead.

HAROLD RUSSELL

PREFACE

THE IMPORTANT THINGS in life do not get done by programs or laws or organizations. They get done by people.

This is a book about some unusual people. A stranger mix of personalities and motivations would be hard to find.

What they produced is peculiarly and completely a product of the Twentieth Century. The ideas they conceived, the knowledge they developed to carry out the ideas, did not exist before this century.

Their work, called rehabilitation for lack of a shorter and better word, has had a profound effect on the lives of millions of disabled people and it will influence the lives of millions not yet born.

For so many of the early rehabilitation leaders, there were the lonely years, when neither the public nor other professionals knew what they were talking about, or cared. There were the building years, when small islands of success had to be carefully cultivated on the way to better understanding and acceptance.

They were not a particularly saintly group. There was even a normal share of rascals. They could, and did, display petty jealousies and magnificent cooperation, sometimes on the same day. There were the brilliant scientific minds, the determined plodders, the sharp executives, the pillars of rectitude, the adroit promoters, the ministering angels.

The notable events, large and small, which marked the development of rehabilitation programs did not occur in isolation. They were a part of the social, industrial, technical and sometimes moral thinking, the general climate and the circumstances, which prevailed in the nation at the time. For this reason I have tried to convey, from time to time, some sense of the changing conditions under which rehabilitation for the disabled emerged and grew.

I realized early that it was not possible to tell this full story, to portray the roles played by every person who helped build the nation's present structure for restoring disabled people to activity and usefulness. That would require several volumes. But I felt that a start must be made now, while the story is still fairly recent and many of the key figures can be consulted. Perhaps other authors will be encouraged to add to the story.

I am much indebted to large numbers of friends, acquaintances and strangers across the country, in public and private agencies and in private life, who responded promptly to my request for factual data and background information used in this book. For special help in a variety of forms, I express my gratitude to these individuals and organizations:

To the Library of Congress and its staff;

To Mr. Donald G. Weiss, Director of Public Relations and Community Education, Dr. Salvatore G. DiMichael, Director, and the library staff of the Institute for the Crippled and Disabled, New York City;

To Mr. Earl Graham, librarian and editor, National Easter Seal Society for Crippled Children and Adults, Chicago;

To Frank E. Mason, retired publisher, Leesburg, Va.;

To my wife Jo, for her frequent help, her unflagging interest and her personal support for an often-bedevilled author;

To Mrs. Cozette Barker of our professional staff for the excellence of her research work in certain phases of the book;

To Mrs. Karyl Luck for her patient and skillful handling of an obstreperous manuscript.

RUSSELL J. N. DEAN

CHAPTER I

A NEW CENTURY

———◆••◆———

THE WORD WAS: Prosperity. Profits were up, employment was high, the iron and steel industry was thriving, the corn crop in Kansas set a record.

Greeting the new 20th Century, the San Francisco *Examiner* said on January 1, 1900: "Never were bank clearings so large. Never within recollection have so few of our people been idle when they have wanted to work." *The New York Times,* analyzing the outlook, editorialized: "Unquestionably to the great body of businessmen the outlook on the threshold of the new year is extremely bright." Some of their optimism flowed from a survey they had done of the nation's Governors, who collectively were convinced that "the country is entering upon a new period of prosperity."

More than two thousand citizens stood in line that day at the White House gates to pay their respects to President and Mrs. William McKinley, and in Albany, N. Y., Governor Theodore Roosevelt held his annual reception for the public at the Executive Chamber.

Boom talk was everywhere, and the word had spread across the seas. The immigrants were coming in growing numbers, mainly from western and middle Europe and the British Isles. In the first year of the century, over 400,000 of them would walk and wait their way through Ellis Island in New York harbor, then turn their faces to a new city, a new land and, they hoped, a new life.

They had reason to dream. Here a man could be his own man, not held fast to the trade and the station in life of his father. Even if the streets were not paved with gold, as some had said, a man could get a job, work hard, save his money and make a fortune. A man could make ten to fifteen dollars a week—and much more if he was a smart, industrious young man—and anyone knows you can raise a family on that kind of money, with free public schools for the kids, eggs at twelve cents a dozen and beer a nickel.

For the professional man, a new age was dawning in medicine. The British surgeon, Joseph Lister, following up on Pasteur's discovery of the bacterial nature of wine-making, had set the scientific world tilting some thirty-five years before by showing that disease was caused by microscopic bacterial organisms, not by "humours" or "rheums" or an over-supply of blood. With his carbolic acid and his bellows, he had convinced more and more skeptics that asepsis could change the practice of surgery and that medicine was really entering a new age of science.

Any child could go to school and get a basic education in the three R's and more. At least, that was the way it was supposed to work, although the noise of protest over the exploitation of child labor in the sweatshops of the garment industry was being heard louder each year. Still, it was hard to argue the point, for public school enrollments had climbed to around 17,000,000 and some 240,000 young people were in college.

There was not much discussion of "communication." People just travelled around and talked and wrote and read and let it go at that. No question about it—there was a lot better chance to be well-informed, with the Post Office handling more than seven billion pieces of mail a year, the railroads carrying passengers over more than sixteen million miles annually, the book publishers bringing out 5,000 new volumes and more than 2,000 daily newspapers reaching over 15,000,000 people each day.

Even that noisy new gadget, the automobile, was catching on, with more than 8,000 of them giving the fidgets to countless horses and their drivers.

Any way you looked at it, this beginning of a new century was a fine time to be alive, for millions of Americans.

But if you were crippled by an accident, or a quirk of birth, or a serious disease, it was not a good time at all.

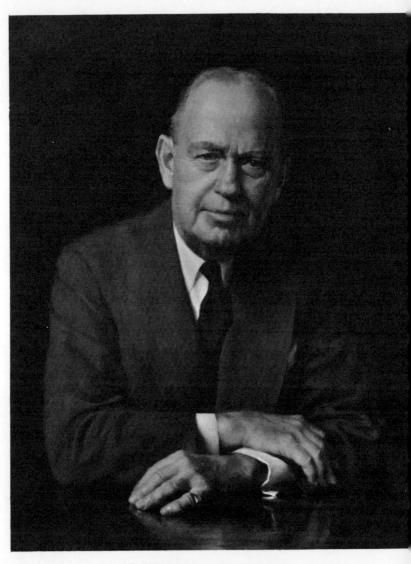

JEREMIAH MILBANK

CHAPTER II

WAR AND POSTWAR

————◆••◆————

OF THE MANY THINGS so peculiarly the product of the Twentieth Century, none is more unique to the time than the ideas and the programs conceived and created to "rehabilitate" disabled people.

In many ways, this approach to an ancient and widespread human problem was a natural outgrowth for a nation which in this century increasingly became committed, even addicted, to the idea of accomplishing all sorts of wonders and solving all manner of problems by concentrating a variety of skills on one objective. This was the story, the method, of industry, of research, of warfare.

It was not easy, in industry, to overcome old ways of doing things and to convince both management and skilled professionals of the virtues of pooling talents in search of a better product.

But compared to the obstacles in efforts for the disabled, industry had it easy. The prospect of increased profits can and did move mountains.

In trying to "sell" a new approach to disability, the only ones who profited were the disabled people and their communities.

It is doubtful that modern methods of dealing with disability could have come along any sooner. Even if the broader concepts had been there—and they were not, except in the most diffuse form—the science and the technology had not arrived. Social theory must always await the tools of social progress.

The beginning of the century was a time when, despite voices to the contrary here and there, a nation lived and rejoiced in the Horatio Alger idea. If you or your parents had lived under the class restrictions of most European societies, you would have embraced Horatio Alger too. Here you could try.

As part of this highly competitive ethic, there were many ways to rationalize the large numbers who did not make the top, or even a view of the top. One of the easiest was to fall back on the ingrained historical attitude toward the "cripple," which either saw the hand of the Lord at work in producing a deformed child or mysterious disease, or which saw no place in the world of work or other normal life for anyone who was "different."

There had been, of course, beginnings, for throughout history there have been men and women who could devote themselves completely to some form of help for the physical and mental victims of a highly imperfect world. By the beginning of the Twentieth Century, a few surgeons had tried some new techniques to provide better "stumps" for those who had lost limbs. Several groups had set up special schools to educate handicapped children. Louis Braille had published his system of dots more than seventy years before, to enable blind persons to read, and a controversy was under way in New York and elsewhere over revisions in his system. The Federal government, back in 1864, had set up Gallaudet College in the nation's capital city to educate young deaf people. Many religious groups, following their centuries-old missions of mercy, were providing havens and other help for many maimed and mentally handicapped people.

Yet the "state of the art" in dealing effectively with disease and injury was, for the most part, primitive. The sulfonamides were unknown and the antibiotics had not yet come along to control infections and thus make rehabilitation both possible and necessary for millions of patients. Artificial limbs were symbolized by the peg legs of such well-known figures as Governor Stuyvesant of New York and Long John Silver of "Treasure Island." Where an artificial leg actually was used, it was a heavy, awkward affair made even more difficult by a poorly-prepared stump and little or no training in its use. More popular and generally better were the crutches available, with one merchant offering, through New York *Times* advertising in 1910, "everyday" maple crutches for $2.50 to $4.00 per pair and gold-trimmed, gem-studded ones for as much as $200.

For the educational needs of the severely handicapped child, the still-evolving public school system rarely accepted the task. Few people asked why, for the prevailing opinion was that such children were best kept out of sight.

For the thousands of workmen severely injured in the rugged phases of America's new industries, there was little recourse except relatives, charity and prayer. The idea of workmen's compensation had been born but the adversary system still prevailed.

In a few places there were developments which, by a combination of chance and good leadership, would survive to take a place in the future of rehabilitation. Before the turn of the century, a group of school girls in Cleveland had formed a club, the "Sunbeam Circle," to help bedfast children in a ward at the old Lakeside Hospital. From this they progressed to a kindergarten for crippled children and then into special education classes. From such a beginning, and in a series of changes over more than half a century, there developed the Cleveland Vocational Guidance and Rehabilitation Services.

In 1902, in Boston's desperately poor South End, a young minister named Edgar J. Helms struggled for better ways to help the poor, the handicapped and other unfortunate people in his community. When he was able to collect clothing and furniture, he never could distribute it in a fair way where it was needed the most. Almost in desperation, he decided that the poor people who came to his Morgan Memorial Chapel should be the ones to sort and mend and clean the clothing, repair the furniture and generally do the work. Then they would earn, on the basis of the work they had done, their fair share of the materials. The plan worked so well that before long, he found it possible to sell part of the collected materials and pay tiny wages to those who had worked.

As the plan caught on in other places, a group in Brooklyn in 1915 named their new program Goodwill Industries.

Such links with the future of rehabilitation were rare in that period. The problems of severe disability not only remained unsolved but unchallenged. Much of the medical, technical, educational and other knowledge the world would need was slowly accumulating; much of the progress in social thinking was underway—but nothing significant had happened to crystallize these elements into either a vision or a plan for the disabled.

There is reason to believe that the chain of events which led to modern rehabilitation concepts was set in motion in the little town of Sarajevo in Bosnia in 1914. There, on June 28, the heir to the Austro-Hungarian empire, Archduke Francis and his wife the Duchess of Hohenberg were assassinated by a young Serbian nationalist. The flame of World War I had been lighted.

The United States watched and waited and hoped that the German war machine would be satisfied with a limited conquest. This was no time for war; a prosperous country found itself caught between its commitments in Europe and its strong isolationist sentiments at home, between its increasingly powerful role on the high seas and its small army.

President Wilson was re-elected in 1916 on a campaign based on keeping the country out of the war. But the sinking of the Lusitania in 1915 and the Sussex in 1916 kept the issue alive, while the German insistence on the right to wage unrestricted submarine warfare was an intolerable challenge to a nation sensitive to its new role as a world power.

It was easy enough to put the ominous war situation aside. There were the new "flickers" with Mary Pickford playing to full houses in "Rebecca of Sunnybrook Farm," and the "vamp," Theda Bara, giving the men quivers and the ladies fits with her performance in "Cleopatra."

And for those who savored their glass of beer or stronger spirits, there was a far more serious crisis in the making than a war: those blue-nose "prohibition" people were about to outlaw a man's right to have a quiet drink.

So despite all the waves of war talk, there was little in the way of preparation-in-depth, and practically none to deal with the one certain aftermath—the disabled soldier.

By the time the United States entered the conflict in 1917, the warring nations in Europe already had gained some experience. In France the government had taken several steps to try to meet some of the need. In the city of Lyons, Mayor Herriot established a training school for the *mutilés de la guerre*. Although simple in concept, the school offered training in a great variety of skilled trades, clerical work, fabrication of artificial limbs, and agriculture, and thus met a practical need for large numbers of disabled veterans. In a limited way, the success of the school, and the establishment of others to take advantage of the Lyons success, helped strengthen the feeling that more should be done for the veterans than a meagre pensioning system.

The British also had developed plans and were able to set a few programs in motion rather early, notably the large center at Roehampton, where private limb makers were assembled to produce the limbs and the government supervised the general operation.

Germany, prepared for war, also had prepared for her veterans, including those disabled in the war. A rather impressive array of facilities and services had been developed in peacetime, for children and adults including the industrially disabled; these immediately became directed to disabled veterans after the war began. Fifty-eight privately-operated facilities for cripples had been established and a large national organization, the German National Federation for the Care of Cripples, had been a leadership organization for many years.

Canada had moved promptly to develop programs too, as had Australia, and it was to be Canada's role to greatly influence and speed the plans of the United States.

In the United States, there was no organized system, or even the elements of a system, for the disabled adult. Several employment bureaus for cripples had been functioning courageously in New York, Boston, Cincinnati and Philadelphia but their size was tiny in relation to need, their support was even smaller, and their resources for training and otherwise preparing the disabled adult for suitable work were zero.

Certainly some impetus, some driving spirit, some focal point was needed to dramatize the need of the United States for a plan to cope with the disability that was certain to arise from participation in the war. As things stood, the country that had hoped to stay out of the war was ill-prepared for the human results of war.

It was in such a situation that Jeremiah Milbank, New York industrialist and philanthropist, moved into the picture. He had been concerned and disturbed, before hostilities, with the sight of so many crippled beggars on the streets of New York, with no practical means of helping them. Now, with a war ahead, there was the further grim outlook—the same lack of facilities for restoring crippled soldiers and sailors when they returned from the war.

It was an unusual and not particularly fashionable cause for a wealthy thirty-year-old to take up. But Mr. Milbank was personally convinced that facilities and services designed especially for the training and rehabilitation of the disabled could help solve one of the nation's widespread human problems. He had read of the early work done in Canada to help returning disabled veterans there and was determined that the United States must make its start at once.

From the outset, Mr. Milbank had some basic ideas about the respective roles of the government and private agencies in developing programs for the disabled, and he remained convinced of these concepts throughout his life. He saw the private agencies pioneering new developments, better techniques and methods, and serving as the point of the spear through research and teaching. He expected the government, with its vaster resources, to see to it that the benefits of all this creative effort were made available to the disabled everywhere.

Accustomed to consulting experts, Mr. Milbank discussed the situation with several people with varied experiences in the problems of the handicapped. Out of these came one relationship which was described in some detail years later by Dr. John Culbert Faries: "For advice Mr. Milbank turned to Dr. Edward T. Devine, Director of the New York School of Philanthropy, whose large experience in the field of social service qualified him to render wise counsel. It was felt that any experience that might be acquired as to the best means for restoring the handicapped civilian to self-supporting activity, even before there were disabled soldiers to be rehabilitated, would be ground gained in solving the problem of the wounded veteran."

"Few public-spirited men, desirous of making a wise investment in welfare work, have been so far-sighted as was Mr. Milbank in choosing to invest his money in a social effort yielding such large dividends in reconstructed lives as work for the handicapped . . ."

"In deciding that this should be his war contribution, Mr. Milbank inaugurated a pioneer work for handicapped persons which not only helped to prepare the way for a constructive program for the rehabilitation of the war cripple, but focused attention upon the duty of the state to assist the civilian cripple to become a self-respecting and self-supporting unit of society."

Dr. Devine was able to bring into this picture two individuals who were experienced in work for crippled children and had an intense interest in the growing problem of disabled adults—Mr. Douglas C. McMurtrie, President of the Federation of Associations for Cripples, and the Federation's Vice-President, Miss Florence C. Sullivan.

In developing his initial steps, Mr. Milbank was convinced that the most effective mechanism under wartime conditions would be the American Red Cross. He went to Washington and discussed his plans with Jesse Jones, Director of Military Relief for the Red Cross. Jones, impressed with the idea, paid a return visit to Mr. Milbank in New York, looked over the specifics of the plans, and later reported to the American Red Cross that this plan should be adopted. Mr. Milbank and Mr. McMurtrie then appeared before the American Red Cross in Washington.

To give substance to his proposal, Mr. Milbank offered to contribute $50,000 toward a rehabilitation facility and to provide a building at the northeast corner of 23rd Street and Fourth Avenue in New York City for this purpose.

In a letter of June 25, 1917, to Eliot Wadsworth, acting chairman of the American Red Cross in Washington, Mr. Milbank formalized his offer. By return mail, Mr. Milbank received formal acceptance of his proposal.

And so, less than three months after the United States' entry into World War I—and one day before the first American soldiers arrived in France—the Red Cross Institution for Crippled Soldiers and Sailors was born.

By midsummer, Dr. Devine and his associates had accomplished a remarkable number and variety of tasks. On August 13, 1917 he reported to the American Red Cross that, in addition to readying the building and numerous other basic chores, he had conducted ". . . a study of peace cripples, *i.e.,* of men who have had amputations performed in New York hospitals since January, 1915, or who as the result of industrial accidents have been known to the Compensation Board of the state Industrial Department. We have obtained definite information concerning over three hundred such cases. The purpose of this inquiry has been to discover the economic effect of particular injuries, to see to what extent men who have suffered these injuries have been able to return to their old occupations or to take up others, and in general to gather any information which would be likely to be useful in dealing with war cripples. We are now analyzing these records and preparing a report on them."

They examined the records of the special Employment Bureau for the Handicapped which had been conducted for

six years (1906 to 1912) by the New York Charity Organization Society.

They sought advice on technical education and other
matters from a variety of experts including those in the
Department of Labor, the National Society for the Promotion of Industrial Education, and among various trade union
officials and vocational education leaders.

Dr. Devine, Mr. McMurtrie and Charles H. Winslow
made a special visit to Canada to observe the work which
had been developed there for their own war disabled veterans. Their studies took them to Quebec, Montreal, Ot-
tawa, and Toronto; Mr. McMurtrie subsequently visited
Winnipeg and Calgary also.

Dr. Devine and Mr. McMurtrie set up a special library
to acquire and catalog technical and other information on
disabled people, with particular reference to the war disabled. Their initial effort provided twice as many titles as
the Library of Congress then listed in its special manuscript
bibliography.

An expert statistician, Dr. I. M. Rubinow, was engaged
to make an actuarial estimate of the number of peace cripples and such estimates as were possible of the probable
number of war crippled who would need vocational rehabilitation. (Dr. Rubinow's preliminary estimates indicated that,
based on the European experience, there probably would be
about fifty thousand permanently disabled veterans each
year for every million soldiers in uniform.)

The results of these comprehensive studies—statistical,
factual and conceptual—formed the guidelines for the establishment of the new institute.

There was a brief interruption of progress in the early
fall. Dr. Devine, assigned by Mr. Milbank to visit France
and other countries as part of the investigation into successful methods, was asked while in Paris to take on an emergency program there in Red Cross relief work. He accepted

and, for a short period, the Institute project was without a program director. Mr. Milbank then persuaded Mr. Mc-Murtrie to accept this new responsibility and McMurtrie became the first Director of what was to become famous as the Institute for the Crippled and Disabled.

The Surgeon General of the Army, Dr. W. C. Gorgas, approved the idea of the new Institute—but with considerable crossing of his fingers. The hero of the conquest of malaria in Panama, in a letter to the Director General of Military Relief of the Red Cross, expressed grave concern that the establishment of such an institute might be followed by others, all of them appealing to the public for funds, with the responsibility of the Federal government to care for disabled veterans being obscured in the process. But after expressing his reservations and doubts, he agreed.

And so a point of reference, a place of technical competence and social dedication, was created to help pave the way for the thousands of disabled men who would come back less than whole from the war, and for the greater thousands of civilian men, women and children who would face the same problems later.

It was an influence that would help in many ways, including the task of writing laws to fashion a national program for veterans. The Congress had acquired some preliminary exposure to the concept of providing special programs for young men, and particularly veterans, in recent years. The National Defense Act passed in 1916 had expressed the policy that soldiers in service should have the benefit of vocational training which would help prepare them for useful work after leaving the service. The following year another new law, the Smith-Hughes Act, had established a Federal-state program to promote and support vocational education and, in the process, created the Federal Board for Vocational Education.

Later that year, amendments to the War Risk Insurance Act made provision for military personnel who were victims of ". . . dismemberment, of injuries to sight or hearing, and of other injuries commonly causing permanent disability . . ." to receive ". . . such course or courses of rehabilitation and vocational training as the United States may provide or procure to be provided." If the person could not make a living for himself while taking such training, he could be continued in service in a special type of enlistment and receive his usual pay and allowances.

Like so many laws, these read better than they worked, particularly for the disabled. By the spring of 1918, the Congress had completed work on another bill, the Vocational Rehabilitation Act, written specifically to meet the problem of the returning disabled veteran. Signed on June 27, it vested the basic authority and responsibility for vocational rehabilitation of veterans in the Federal Board for Vocational Education. So the War Department, after winning control over the training of disabled soldiers through the 1916 National Defense Act (and then doing very little about it) had lost the big battle for control of such programs for the disabled of World War I.

In trying to set such a program in motion, the administrative and jurisdictional snarls were so prevalent that the war was over before some of them were untangled.

From the time the new law was passed in June until early December of that year, rehabilitation personnel of the Federal Board were not permitted to contact any disabled veterans in military hospitals. The Surgeon General contended that disabled men should be treated and restored to duty for non-combat functions, and therefore should not be exposed to ideas from non-military personnel. By the time this barrier was lowered, several thousand disabled men had been discharged from service without ever knowing that the government intended to help them.

Although the Federal Board for Vocational Education had responsibility for conducting the vocationl rehabilitation program for veterans, only the Bureau of War Risk Insurance (a completely separate and independent agency) could make the determination that the veteran was eligible. It was the Bureau which received and tried to process the claims for disability compensation—and the Bureau quickly became inundated with far more claims than they could process. Disabled veterans waited both for compensation (on which many of them depended entirely to subsist during the post-discharge period) and for vocational rehabilitation services.

Throughout the furor that persisted, the Federal Board for Vocational Education retained, for the most part, a posture of administrative responsibility and was generally credited with doing everything possible under an impossible situation. It was July 11, 1919—two weeks after the Treaty of Versailles was signed to formally end World War I—before the Congress changed the law to place the responsibility for determining eligibility for vocational rehabilitation on the Federal Board for Vocational Education. There remained a host of problems—the development of program, the hiring and training of competent staffs, the setting up of field organizations and the development of working relationships with other public and private agencies. A combination of a better basic law, plus the end of the war itself, enabled the Federal Board to finally begin moving aggressively and more successfully.

But the combination of legal and administrative roadblocks, complaints of delay in services, opposition from veterans organizations and others, mistakes made in the process of experimenting—all these combined to exert strong pressures for change. In August of 1921, President Harding signed a law transferring the Board's Veterans Rehabilitation Division (along with the Bureau of War Risk Insurance, the Pension Bureau and the veterans' health functions of the Public Health Service) to a new agency, the Veterans Bureau.

In the long perspective, the tribulations of the Federal Board and the fate of the nation's first public vocational rehabilitation program for veterans were of less consequence to the future of rehabilitation in the United States than some of the other developments which had sprung from the pressures of war.

For one thing, the military hospitals responded more successfully to the acute and restorative needs of their hospitalized patients than in any previous episode in military history. Without aircraft for quick evacuation, without antibiotics, without a medical answer to the ravages of the mustard and phosgene gases, without either the scientific or physical resources to deal aggressively with "shell shock," the military medical system still provided the best medical care any group of veterans had ever received.

Plans were made for three "Reconstruction Hospitals" to receive the seriously disabled veterans, along with the extensive resources of Walter Reed Hospital in Washington, D. C. Of the three, only one—Reconstruction Hospital No. 3 at Colonia, N. J.—was opened and used. It became, however, an important institution of the period, both because of the advanced rehabilitation work done there and because it permitted one of the creative physicians of the time, Dr. Fred H. Albee, to launch many of his ideas in restoring the disabled.

Reconstruction Hospital No. 3 functioned for only sixteen months, closing in October of 1919, but it accomplished much. More than six thousand disabled veterans had been treated and Dr. Albee's concepts and methods for providing an array of services, to reduce or remove the disability and to prepare the patient for resumption of a useful civilian life, had left their mark on rehabilitation history and practice.

The Army Surgeon General and his staff did more: they encouraged and helped establish some of the rehabilitative approaches and the professional groups that were destined to become vital parts of future rehabilitation programs.

One of these was occupational therapy. The idea was not new; it had been born many years before and nurtured by some of the early leaders like Susan Tracy, Eleanor Clarke Slagle and Dr. William Rush Dunton, Jr. There was even an infant organization, formed three weeks before war was declared, which would later become the American Occupational Therapy Association.

The OT organization in 1917 reached out to one of the most interesting personalities of the time, and for many years to come, when they named Frank B. Gilbreth an honorary member. Frank Gilbreth and his wife Lillian at that time were in the early and trail-blazing stage of developing the concepts and methods of time-motion studies to promote greater efficiency in all sorts of industrial, commercial and other activities. They became interested in trying to adapt some of their techniques to solving problems for handicapped people—an interest which persisted throughout most of their lives, and which had an obvious appeal for occupational therapists in their work with patients. As outstanding figures in time study engineering, they became well known to their own profession and in much of industrial engineering; as contributors to work for the handicapped, they became known to many people in rehabilitation; but it remained for son Frank Gilbreth, Jr. and daughter Ernestine Gilbreth Carey to make the world familiar with the rollicking Gilbreth family in their books *Cheaper by the Dozen* and *Belles on Their Toes* and the latest by Frank Gilbreth, Jr., *Time Out for Happiness.*

The first proposals of Miss Slagle for providing occupational therapy for hospitalized soldiers met a wall of opposition. But she persisted and by 1918, Surgeon General Gorgas not only agreed to the appointment of "reconstruction aides" but later called for a thousand aides at once and four thousand more within six months. This was a larger order than the OT's or anyone else could fill but they went into action, establishing training centers to provide six-week courses and staffing Army hospitals as fast as the graduates could be produced.

Another group of "reconstruction aides"—these the forerunners of today's physical therapists—was transformed from a good idea to an established group as a result of the Army's emergency steps to serve the injured and ill veteran. Mainly through the efforts of Colonel Joel E. Goldsthwait and Colonel E. G. Brackett, the Women's Auxiliary Aids was organized in the Surgeon General's Office late in 1917. By 1918 the title was changed to "Reconstruction Aides," with Dr. Frank E. Granger in charge, and the unit made a part of the Division of Physical Reconstruction.

To meet the pressing demands for more physical therapists to serve the growing lists of disabled soldiers, a course was organized at Walter Reed Army Hospital in Washington and the help of a number of colleges with departments of physical education was secured to conduct emergency courses to train more "reconstruction aides." By 1919, Miss Mary McMillen, one of the early group working with the Army and in the training efforts, became Supervisor of Reconstruction Aides in Physiotherapy, in the Office of the Surgeon General. By the war's end, nearly eight hundred had served the Army, three hundred of them overseas. Their success led to the formation in 1920 of the first professional organization, the American Women's Therapeutic Association, which evolved into the present organization, the American Physical Therapy Association.

There were many spin-offs from the work of the military forces, some of which not only began "movements" but also began some cross-fertilizing among people and places. One of the reconstruction aides, Elizabeth Upham, (later Mrs. Carl Henry Davis) returned to her native Milwaukee and persuaded her fellow members in the Junior League to support the opening of a program of occupational therapy and physical therapy for handicapped children. From that small original effort in a cottage on the grounds of Columbia Hospital, there developed over the years today's Curative Workshop of Milwaukee.

According to Dr. Henry H. Kessler, Miss Upham did more. Writing in "Rehabilitation Literature" in 1965, he recalled that "Occupational therapy was having a great boom in England and Canada and rumors of its advantages reached down into many of the military hospitals. As a matter of fact, it was Miss Elizabeth G. Upham, a director of a college art department who was interested in social work, who sought to gain Mr. Milbank's interest in establishing an occupational therapy program in the United States."

The Army also had supported the establishment of another Red Cross war service facility, this aimed at serving veterans blinded in the war. "Evergreen," the Red Cross Institute for the Blind at Baltimore, became better known as one of the forerunners of the American Foundation for the Blind than for its work with World War I veterans. It remained for such established leaders as the Perkins Institution and Massachusetts School for the Blind in Boston, and the New York Institute for the Blind, along with the state schools for the blind, and the American Association of Workers for the Blind, to provide the basis for long-range growth and improvement of educational and other service programs for blind people.

By the time the armistice was signed ending hostilities

in November, 1918, the Red Cross Institution for Crippled and Disabled Men was deeply engaged in providing training for a growing number of disabled. Fewer veterans than expected were among them, because of the administrative impasse that existed between the government agencies, but the number of civilian crippled mounted steadily. Training courses were provided in drafting, motion picture projection, jewelry manufacture, oxyacetylene welding, job printing and artificial limb making.

The Institute promoted certain ideas that in coming years found their way into basic rehabilitation precepts. One was that, wherever possible, medical and surgical services should be available to reduce or eliminate the disability. For this, the Institute arranged with clinics and hospitals in New York to provide such services wherever the prognosis was favorable.

Another was that the disabled person should be brought into an active rehabilitation program as promptly as possible after injury. To encourage this in practice, a social worker was added to the Institute staff in 1918 and regularly visited the wards of New York hospitals to locate patients with disabling conditions and try to arrange for their early referral to the Institute.

Believing that training must result in placement in a suitable job, the Institute conducted a special placement service. It went beyond the needs of its own trainees; it welcomed all disabled who were having difficulties securing a job. In the first ten months of its work, the Institute registered more than 700 disabled and placed 620 of them.

Perhaps the most important long-range pioneering was done in educating hundreds of groups, and the general public, to the need and the benefits of special programs to rehabilitate the disabled. It was Mr. Milbank's aim that the Red Cross Institute for the Crippled and Disabled do more than serve the disabled; it must function as a rallying point for the whole effort to make known the plight of the disabled and the need to do something constructive about it.

For this, he had the right man in McMurtrie, who must have been one of the busiest men of his day.

From the Institute's new home at 23rd Street and Fourth Avenue in Manhattan (which originally had housed the College of Physicians and Surgeons) there began flowing a stream of educationl and promotional programming that reached into hundreds of cities across the country and into the lives of countless disabled men, women and children.

A publicity service began operating early in 1918. Articles were prepared for trade journals and other publications.

A news service was operated which covered not only the major New York papers but also several of those still-new systems, the newspaper syndicates.

Material on rehabilitation of the disabled went direct to a mailing list of more than a thousand newspapers.

A public speakers' bureau was organized, including training for volunteer speakers, which brought the story to over three hundred meetings and their thousands of listeners.

A series of eighty-five lantern slide presentations was prepared, plus twenty-two reels of motion pictures, used by speakers and made available to groups to help explain the story, the need and the plans.

A series of leaflets was produced and more than seven million of them distributed. One was translated into French, Italian, German, Swedish, Danish, Spanish, Polish, Hungarian, Greek and Yiddish.

The Institute became the publication office of an illustrated magazine, *Carry On,* published by the American Red Cross for the Office of the Surgeon General of the Army.

One of the results of this crescendo of activity was the convening of the first international conference on rehabilitation of the disabled in this country. The conference, held March 18–23, 1919, was jointly developed and sponsored by the Red Cross Institute for Crippled and Disabled Men, the Federal Board for Vocational Education, the Red Cross Institute for the Blind, and the Office of the Surgeon General of the Army. Delegates came from France, Belgium, Italy, Great Britain and Canada. Technical sessions were held in the Waldorf Astoria and the general sessions in Carnegie Hall. On Sunday, March 23, for the closing affair, a great mass meeting was held in the Hippodrome attended by thousands, including hundreds of disabled soldiers and sailors brought by the Red Cross ambulances and given the best seats.

The Honorable Charles Evans Hughes introduced the principal speakers, two of whom had achieved remarkable careers in spite of their severe disabilities. One was the Honorable Michael Dowling of Minnesota, the other Judge Quentin D. Corley of Dallas. It was Dowling who held the throng spellbound with a story—his own story—of a sheepherder boy caught in a Minnesota blizzard and left so frozen that he lost both legs below the knee, his left hand and all the fingers and part of the thumb on his right. But the fourteen-year-old boy, helped by the County Poor Commissioners, went on to college and to a distinguished career in business and the State Legislature.

At the end of the speech, with the crowd applauding wildly, Justice Hughes remarked, "That was the finest American speech I ever heard!"

The British Red Cross invited Mr. Dowling and Judge Corley to appear in England and they agreed. But before leaving, Dowling journeyed across the Hudson River to join McMurtrie and others in testifying in support of a bill before the New Jersey legislature—a bill proposing to establish a vocational rehabilitation program for disabled civilians in that state. He thus became a part of the history of one of the first state-operated rehabilitation programs in the country.

Before the big international conference closed, the Federal Board for Vocational Education proposed that twenty-five men and women be selected to take a special training course at the Red Cross Institute for Crippled and Disabled Men.

When this was agreed to, Jeremiah Milbank underwrote the costs for the trainees, then added a post-course study trip through Canada to acquaint them first-hand with the work being done there for disabled soldiers.

In a way, the conclusion of the conference was both an end and a beginning. It had formalized much of the fervor, the pressures that had gone into this country's belated and hectic effort to literally throw together some kind of program to meet the needs of veterans returning disabled from the war. With the fighting ended and with the formalities of the Treaty of Versailles only three months ahead, it was the end of a period.

But it was, as they hoped, a beginning for the idea that disabled people—veterans and non-veterans, men, women and children—must have specialized rehabilitation programs to rescue them from social and vocational oblivion. It was the beginning of the idea that government must accept an active role in seeing that this is done, and encourage and help private organizations conduct programs.

Most important, comprehensive rehabilitation for the disabled had moved beyond the idea stage. A beginning had been made.

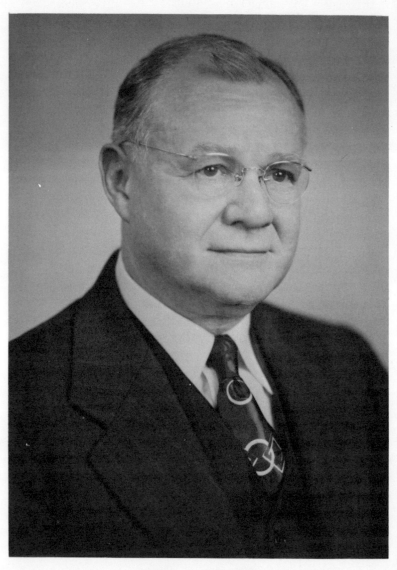

JOHN A. KRATZ

CHAPTER III

TRIAL FLIGHT

On June 2, 1920 a tragically disabled President of the United States signed into law the first Federal Act to provide vocational rehabilitation services for disabled civilians.

Woodrow Wilson had encouraged laws and programs for his disabled veterans and had signed the disabled veterans' rehabilitation law. Now the Commander-in-Chief became one of them.

Unlike the disabled veterans from the ranks, he bore no scars when the war was over, only an overpowering weariness that he would not accept. There was the treaty to be negotiated and signed at Versailles—and there was the League of Nations to be nurtured as the hope against future wars.

He had first become ill on April 3, 1919 with what his doctors described as influenza but which many people later believed was the first of his "little strokes." But he proceeded with the treaty negotiations.

On his return in early July, he plunged into a heavy schedule of speeches, reports to Congress, meetings—all to try to build support for United States membership in the

League of Nations. To arouse wide public interest, he started on a national speaking tour. When his doctor, his wife and others insisted he was too ill for such a trip, he was quoted as saying: "I do not want to do anything foolhardy, but the League of Nations is now in its crisis and if it fails, I hate to think of what will happen to the world. You must remember that I, as Commander-in-Chief, was responsible for sending our soldiers to Europe. In the crucial test of the trenches they did not turn back—and I cannot turn back now. I cannot put my personal safety, my health, in the balance against my duty."

On September 25, 1919, after leaving Pueblo, Colorado, he collapsed. The rest of the trip was cancelled and the Presidential party returned to Washington. On October 2 he suffered a stroke which paralyzed his left side. He would, almost by personal courage, see his term of office through to the end but he would fill that office as the world's most powerful hemiplegic.

For the lesser-known victims of disability, the impetus of the World War drive for veterans' rehabilitation programs now was being concentrated on the needs of the non-veteran —the industrial accident cases, the farm workers and all the others who found their lives engulfed by a disabling condition and the barriers it raised.

Among the many "post-war readjustments," the American Red Cross was divesting itself of its special wartime activities. On the first observance of Armistice Day in 1919, the Red Cross Institute for Crippled and Disabled Men became a private organization, the Institute for Crippled and Disabled Men (and later would be simply the Institute for the Crippled and Disabled). Now it would have to prove itself again as an independent facility and the start was auspicious, with a Board of Trustees bearing such names as Mrs. August Belmont, Walter E. Hope and Miss Ethel Mc-

Lean, and with Samuel M. Greer as President. The pioneers were still there, with Jeremiah Milbank as Treasurer, Douglas McMurtrie as Secretary and Florence Sullivan as Vice-President.

In various places, small events were taking place which would assume large proportions in the coming decades. In Elyria, Ohio, a small group of people interested in crippled children formed a new organization and elected Edgar E. Allen as the first President of the Ohio Society for Crippled Children. Their accomplishments that year didn't startle anyone and they were a long way from the day of Easter Seals—but something important had been started.

In 1920 a fun-and-frolic group decided to tackle something more serious. For years the Shriners had enjoyed themselves at meetings and public events, an ebullient caravan of business and professional men at play. But one of their leaders, W. Freeland Kendrick, Potentate of Lu Lu Temple in Philadelphia, insisted that the Shriners should embrace something more tangible, more responsive to human need. Specifically, he wanted the Shriners to build and operate a hospital for crippled children. After he became Imperial Potentate in 1919, the crippled children's hospital idea became an internal issue; there was strong opposition from many parts of the leadership. At their convention in 1920, it looked for a while as though the opposition would carry the day—until Forrest Adair, head of the Scottish Rite bodies in Atlanta, made his famous "bubbles" speech. The opposition collapsed and the Shriners would have their crippled children's hospital. They would continue their pursuit of fun but the hospital commitment would grow to several hospitals, all of them, in the words of Fred Van Deventer ". . . a gift from men with merry hearts and reverent minds."

In Massachusetts, a limited program for those disabled

covered by Workmen's Compensation had been authorized by the legislature in 1918. Now other states were facing the same set of questions. In the one year of 1919, eight states passed laws providing some type of rehabilitation program for the disabled under State auspices: Illinois, Minnesota, Nevada, New Jersey, North Dakota, Oregon, Pennsylvania and Rhode Island. California passed a law that year but it was taken to court on constitutional grounds and ruled invalid. Early in 1920, two more states—New York and Virginia—joined the "movement." No two state laws were alike, and the provisions for coverage, services and other features varied greatly. Some of the programs were not yet in operation. Yet the states had accepted a role in the problem of disability and a willingness to take beginning steps to deal with it.

For the Federal role, the scene had been set, the commitments made, in the process of arriving at a law for the rehabilitation of veterans.

The story of disability and what could be done about it through rehabilitation programs had been before the legislators and the public.

The extent of serious disability and what it was doing to the lives of shockingly large numbers of Americans had been made clear.

Perhaps most important of all, many Senators and Congressmen, in the process of refusing to include non-veterans along with veterans in the first vocational rehabilitation law, had made commitments to take care of the needs of disabled non-veterans once the "doughboys'" legislation was enacted.

When the first bill was introduced in the fall of 1918 by Congressman William B. Bankhead of Alabama (and a week later by Senator Hoke Smith of Georgia), there was support from several sources.

Two witnesses before the Congressional committees, urging changes in the bill, were pleading for a broad rehabilitation program—one so far ahead of its time that it is doubtful whether the Congress or very many other people really comprehended what they were saying.

One was Douglas McMurtrie, emissary of Jeremiah Milbank and Director of the Red Cross Institute for Crippled and Disabled Men in New York. He pointed to the need for considering the many factors which constitute the problems of disabled people—the frequent need for surgical or other treatment for the disability itself, the social and counselling needs, the practical money problems of those who had no way to live while undertaking a training program, the highly individual character of artificial limb making and fitting and training. He recommended definitions of "disabled persons" and of "rehabilitation" which would be broad and flexible, so that virtually all persons needing services and having prospects for ultimate employment could be served by the proposed Federal-state program.

The committees accepted his definitions, but not his vision of a comprehensive program.

The other forward-looking witness was Lt. Col. Harry E. Mock of the Office of the Army Surgeon General. As a medical man with a background in industrial medicine, and with the benefit of much recent wartime experience in developing programs for disabled veterans, he urged the committees not to limit the service largely to vocational training but to authorize medical and surgical services to eliminate or modify the disability wherever possible, and to provide a variety of other services where needed.

Colonel Mock's proposals were articulate and clear but in vain.

A seasoned politician could have foretold the outcome of these or any other efforts to expand the bills: the Con-

gress was not about to authorize a bigger and better vocational rehabilitation program for disabled non-veterans than
they had just finished authorizing for disabled veterans—not
with the veterans' organizations growing in membership and
strength as hundreds of thousands of soldiers and sailors
shed their uniforms and came streaming into civilian life.

However, the constrictions on the program were, more
than anything else, the product of the time in which the program was born.

The idea that the Federal government might involve
itself in a medical care system for veterans (beyond what
the military services could provide) was radical. Only now,
after the war, was the government beginning to make some
limited provisions for the post-discharge hospital care of
wounded and disabled veterans, and this had evoked much
protest.

Along with this, the choice of an administering agency
—the Federal Board for Vocational Education—while logi-
cal in most ways, eliminated any chance that Congress would
trust such an obviously non-medical and still-new agency to
initiate any sort of medical service program. In fact, by the
time the rehabilitation bill was in its decisive stages in the
Congress, the Federal Board already was under fire for its
handling of the veterans' programs.

Further strengthening the conservative view that a simple program of familiar services aimed at job preparation
was best, the Congress still had serious reservations about
any sort of Federal grant-in-aid programs to the states, despite having agreed to some. It was all right for the states to
do all sorts of things, on their own initiative and funds, as
long as the Federal government did not get involved. One
of the main points of opposition to the vocational rehabilitation bill for civilians was the charge that it invaded states
rights. This charge, on any bill, was enough to sound the

call to many legislators who, like the framers of the Constitution, had an ingrained fear that an ambitious central government might some day dominate the states and thus control the American governmental system. It was with this objection that Senator William H. King of Utah and others belabored the bill.

The criticisms did not rest on this point alone nor were they confined to the 1918 bills, which cleared the Senate and House committees but were not passed in either body.

When the new Congress convened in 1919, it was a Republican-controlled Congress but the sponsors of rehabilitation legislation were the same—and so were the main problems and objections.

The bills were blasted as socialistic, impractical, unconstitutional, Bolshevist, a waste of money, visionary and paternalistic.

They were blessed as a humanitarian measure, a step to conserve needed workers, a good investment in people and the principle of self-support, a way to reduce beggary and the poor farms, and a simple measure to provide equal treatment of the disabled and able-bodied in preparing for useful work.

And, as usual, some legislators paid very little attention at all.

The legislation might have been stalled to death, as it nearly was on several occasions, if it had not had skillful, experienced and determined men handling it.

In the Senate, Senator Hoke Smith had decided some time before that there should be a program for disabled civilians. His experience with the Smith-Hughes Vocational Education Act came into play but he had more qualifications than that. He was an experienced politician—former Governor of Georgia, powerful debater and speaker, former Cabinet officer who knew something about the Federal agencies "downtown." Educated by his father, he had been a lawyer, a newspaper editor and owner, and a political power in his state. An influential figure on and off the Senate floor, Hoke Smith usually got what he wanted.

In the House, the Bankhead member of the original team introduced his bill again but, with the Republicans in charge, a new Chairman of the House Education Committee, Simeon D. Fess of Ohio, decided to make a few changes and introduce his own bill.

So now it was Democrat Smith and Republican Fess—and the two were as different as two men could be. The scholarly Fess had worked his way up from life on an Ohio farm to become a teacher, a college professor of American history, dean of a law school, university president and an editor. Elected to Congress, he was a highly educated midwest conservative yet he consistently showed a concern about people, probably a reflection of his own early struggles and his strong belief in education as a means to a social end.

Despite opposition that sometimes became caustic in both the House and the Senate, the bills passed both houses and by May 1920, the Congress agreed on a final measure.

On June 2, 1920, President Wilson signed it into law as Public Law 236, 66th Congress—and the nation had its first national commitment to using rehabilitation programs to restore disabled civilians.

This not only was the best bill that could be passed; it was a fairly good bill in light of the situation. With a Presidental election ahead in a few months, with Republicans in control of the Congress and a Democrat in the White House, it was rather remarkable that a Republican Senate would pass a Democrat's (Smith's) bill, and that a Democrat (Bankhead) would help pass a Republican's (Fess') bill in the House. The bill, like much domestic legislation at that time, presented no political questions for President Wilson, partly because it certainly would not enter into campaign issues in the fall, and partly because the President's physical condition was so poor that his family and party friends refused to let his name be presented for renomination.

The public generally and the press paid little attention to this latest addition to the statute books.

It was a lot more fun to go to the motion pictures and see Mary Pickford with her new show "Pollyanna" or down the street to see Charlie Chaplin's newest one, "The Kid." John Barrymore was doing "Dr. Jekyll and Mr. Hyde" and the other movies were making a lot of names famous, names like Douglas Fairbanks, Eric von Stroheim, Lillian Gish, Lionel Barrymore, Wallace Reid, Gloria Swanson and many others.

But outside the movie houses, the men were having a bad time. The amendment to the Constitution giving women the vote had gone into effect and many men (and some women) were convinced that the American government would go to hell in a basket once the women started to vote.

To make it worse, the national prohibition law was now in effect and a man could not even get a decent drink to take his mind off these and other troubles. There were "prohibition agents" all over the place, the racketeers were blossoming into the rum running business, and many of the brewers still had not mastered the trick of producing legal "near beer" that was potable. Doctors frequently found themselves pestered with "patients" who mainly wanted a prescription for some legally-dispensed bonded whiskey.

Many people were feeling the effects of unemployment, with the war plants largely closed and too little industry appearing to replace them. Many thousands of soldiers and sailors had gone off to war too young to gain any job experience, so they were poorly prepared to compete in the scramble for post-war jobs.

As the 1920 Presidential election neared, the Republicans had reason to be confident. They held the great advantage of being the party in control of Congress; they had the negative advantage of a President who had promised to keep the country out of war and could not, and who was too ill and disabled to help the party effectively, let alone lead it.

The Democrats, unable to shake the "war party" label, tried. They went to Ohio for a Presidential candidate—Ohio, home of popular Republican Presidents like McKinley and Taft—and nominated Governor James M. Cox. For his running mate, there was a young man from New York, not too well known outside the East, named Franklin D. Roosevelt.

From the hot, sweaty sessions and the "smoke-filled rooms" of their Chicago convention, the tired Republican delegates finally nominated another Ohioan, Senator Warren G. Harding. For the Vice-Presidency, they chose an even less known personality, Calvin Coolidge of Vermont.

The election of Harding to the Presidency, his death three years later, and the subsequent terms of Coolidge, were of concern to the young federal-state rehabilitation program only because they presented a difficult eight-year period in government administration. It was a program created by the signature of a disabled President, followed by a President who would not finish his first term in office, followed by a President whose views on Federal responsibility and Federal spending were matched only by the brevity of his speech.

(One of the stories told by Mrs. Coolidge was about the Washington hostess who said, "Oh, Mr. Coolidge, you are so silent. But you must talk to me. I made a bet today that I could get more than two words out of you."

"You lose," replied Coolidge.)

So, the rehabilitation program quickly developed its own leaders. Those few states having their own vocational rehabiltation laws were elated, for the new Federal rehabilitation law meant that now there would be some Federal interest and help. It meant there would be Federal funds to begin serving the disabled, and the prestige and precedent of a Federal law to help convince state legislatures that this new rehabilitation idea was a good one. Now it would be possible to elicit more interest and more funds from state legislatures, from state workmen's compensation agencies and other sources.

There was only one thing wrong with the state rehabilitation group: there were so very, very few of them.

But a beginning had to be made—and it was. Dr. Charles A. Prosser and his staff in the Federal Board of Vocational Education began work at once, calling in state directors and securing their advice and taking advantage of their experience so far. Some sort of record must have been established in getting on with a new Federal law, for the first *Bulletin* on vocational rehabilitation was issued some three months after the Federal law was passed, giving states initial guidance on concepts and how to proceed in carrying out this new Federal-state cooperative program.

In the fall, a key figure moved on-stage in this fledgeling Federal-state effort. On October 16, 1920, John A. Kratz joined the staff of the Federal Board for Vocational Education, first as a "regional agent" and later that year as Chief of the Vocational Rehabilitation Division of the Board. Mr. Kratz, recently come to the Federal government from several years of experience as a college teacher, quickly displayed a talent for working easily and effectively with the state administrators and for learning the sometimes devious and obscure ways of Federal administration. The developmental work proceeded without delays and, by the early spring of 1921, the Federal staff had reached a total of six people, including such early leaders as Tracy Copp, Frank J.

Clayton, Frederic G. Elton, Lewis H. Carris and Frank Harrison.

The whole apparatus for such a program—the agreement upon principles and policies, the development of program objectives, the consideration of state staffing needs, the distribution and management of Federal funds as well as the requirement upon state funds, a reporting system and the other elements of a unified program—were worked out in detail by Mr. Kratz' unit and the state officials.

Certainly they were not plagued with questions of what to do with the distribution of a large Federal appropriation. For the fiscal year 1921, now nearly ended, the appropriation was $750,000 and for the coming year, when the agencies already organized could expect to begin operating at something approaching their capacities, the total Federal funds amounted to $1 million. These Federal amounts, plus equal amounts required to be furnished by the states, would not rehabilitate a large number of disabled people but they would give this still-experimental program a chance to start.

In trying to carry out some constructive work for the disabled, the state officials had their job cut out for them. The new Federal law did not permit use of Federal funds to provide medical or surgical or hospital care, so there was no opportunity to remove or reduce the disability. The state agencies could not use the funds to pay the living expenses of their handicapped clients while undergoing rehabilitation. Federal money was not available to the state to serve blind persons or the mentally retarded or the mentally ill.

For many of the state officials, the working climate at home was not very inspiring. Many of the state departments of education were heavily influenced by an underlying fear of Federal aid to education. This was compounded in the case of the rehabilitation agencies, which not only functioned within the educational hierarchy but were part of the vocational education functions in the state—and most of the state education departments were not particularly enthusiastic about supporting their own vocational education programs, let alone this new addition to the picture.

Yet the program did move steadily ahead into the Twenties. As always, leadership appears when the need is urgent and into this need came names like Oscar M. Sullivan of Minnesota, W. F. Faulkes of Wisconsin and Dr. R. M. Little of New York. Dr. Little had been closely involved with the broad problem of disability for many years through his work with the U. S. Employees Compensation Commission and had been a strong supporter and effective witness when the vocational rehabilitation bills were before the Congress.

There were people like R. C. (Tommy) Thompson who worked in the early programs of three states (Georgia, South Carolina and Maryland) and was the originator of two of those state programs. There was Marlow Perrin of Ohio, S. S. Riddle of Pennsylvania and R. L. Bynum of Virginia. From the south the leaders were T. C. (Terry) Foster of Alabama, Homer L. Stanton of North Carolina and Sam Woods of Mississippi. The early program in New Jersey was headed by Joseph D. Spitz and in Nebraska, J. R. Jewell.

The vision displayed by some of these men is, in retrospect, remarkable. Oscar Sullivan probably was the first American, certainly in vocational rehabilitation, to suggest a national system of disability insurance along the lines of present-day Social Security disability benefits. In an article in the U. S. Labor Department's "Monthly Labor Review" in 1920, he discussed the advantages and problems of the Minnesota rehabilitation program, pointing out that, although the program could not furnish medical restorative service or artificial appliances or money for maintenance, much of this need was met for many disabled clients through the programs of workmen's compensation; others who were "railroad cases" had similar benefits.

But he went on to observe: "For the other cases, the victims of private accidents and disease, the ideal method would be another resort to the social insurance idea, namely, to provide in a universal health-insurance act limited specific indemnities for such cases. Creation of a public relief fund now would only serve to put off the day when the question would be met properly, and prolong treatment by public charity of a program that should be cured by social insurance."

Mr. Sullivan was not a great believer in surveys, at least as a launching pad for such a new program. Noting that "The Minnesota Division has not inaugurated its work by launching a survey," he gave several reasons—a limited appropriation which could be better spent on services to disabled clients; employers who were already overburdened with surveys; and his own plan to accrue information through a combination of the agency's own work plus the regular surveys conducted by the state's factory inspectors of the Department of Labor.

One of the problems he foresaw remains a problem today: "One of the biggest tasks ahead of the Division is to educate employers to give disabled persons a chance. The Division can and will undertake this, while a regular employment service would probably be unwilling or unable to do so. Many employers still have an idea that insurance companies will raise their rates if they hire handicapped persons. Such an act was made illegal in Minnesota by the 1919 legislature, but it takes time for the information to spread. It is felt, however, that the bulk of the indisposition to hire impaired persons is due to an underestimate of their capacity. Only a prolonged and vigorous campaign of education will overcome this."

It was W. F. Faulkes, director of the Wisconsin state program, who contributed much of the thoughtful planning which went into the development of the early program and into its later stages. With a background in vocational education and a knowledge of the workings of workmen's compensation at that time, he strove to "sell" the concept that vocational rehabilitation should not be limited to the victims of industrial accidents and that to avoid this pitfall, the state agency should not be administratively located within the state Industrial Accident Commissions. He stressed the large numbers of crippled children coming into the employment years annually who had no means of preparing themselves for useful work and responsible lives, and he urged that schools and special education programs do something about this, so that the rehabilitation agencies would be better able to cope with the problem as the disabled children matured.

The early leaders in work for the blind also were beginning to appear. Out of the annual conference of the American Association of Workers for the Blind in 1921 there came a determination to try to establish a national organization for the blind. A group consulted with Major M. C. Migel, a well known philanthropist who already had demonstrated much interest in the problems of blindness. Major Migel underwrote the expenses for the first three years of such a new organization and, on February 1, 1923, the American Foundation for the Blind opened its first offices in New York City. The first officers and staff were to become familiar names in the long history of work for blind people, with Major Migel accepting the presidency, Dr. Joseph C. Nate serving as the Director-General of the new Foundation, and with Dr. Robert B. Irwin as Director of Research and Education. Charles B. Hayes was named Director of Information and Publicity, and Editor of the *Outlook for the Blind*. It was to be Dr. Irwin's destiny to become the Executive Director in 1929 and to lead the Foundation through some of its most formative and successful years.

Among the enthusiastic supporters of the American Foundation for the Blind from its beginnings were Helen Keller and her teacher Anne Sullivan Macy. In the early years, Helen Keller conducted a series of mass meetings across the country to build up what was to be called the Helen Keller Endowment Fund—meetings which made thousands of friends for the new organization. She would later serve as Counselor of National and International Affairs and become a powerful force in promoting Federal and state legislation for the blind.

There were other quiet beginnings which, like the AFB, had nothing to do with the passage of laws and little in common with the public rehabilitation program except the shared impetus of a world war. In Los Angeles, a young orthopedist was about to set forth on a remarkable career of service to the disabled. Back from military duty in 1919, Dr. C. L. Lowman had found that his friend and former patient Mrs. Phoebe Taylor Brockway and her League for Crippled Children were moving his tiny clinic from its home in a small frame house into larger quarters—this time in a converted stable. But this was only the first step in a larger plan. By early 1922, Dr. Lowman and his associates were installed in the first new building—the first of many to come —of the Orthopaedic Hospital of Los Angeles. Dr. Lowman would become an outstanding figure in surgical procedures for disabled children and adults; an exponent, with physical therapist Susan Roen, of therapeutic pools and other hydrology methods for the disabled; a teacher, researcher and clinician; an advisor to the American Occupational Therapy Association, the American Physical Therapy Association, and the California State Bureau of Rehabilitation. He would hold high office in his own professional associations in orthopedic surgery. But perhaps his greatest skill would be his capacity to inspire enthusiasm and dedication among the thousands of professionals, volunteers and civic groups who responded to his leadership.

Another kind of leadership, another set of skills, was called for in Washington if the young Federal-state program was to survive beyond its tenuous beginnings. It was John A. Kratz who rose to this task.

As "The Chief" in the formative years and for many years after, he brought to the program exactly the sort of leadership that was required for the time and the situation. The program ideas, the means of testing them, the political lines to powerful people in the states and Federal government, the direct contacts with the disabled—these and other strengths lay with the state directors of rehabilitation. The fate of the program rested on the ability of the Federal leadership to bring these state officials together tightly in common cause.

John Kratz did this in remarkable fashion, serving more as "chairman" than as policy-maker, more as devoted coordinator than as rule-maker. As a result he was trusted, supported and admired by the state directors, so that the "team approach" in vocational rehabilitation began with its administration.

To these qualities he added a capacity to learn and use effectively the techniques of bureaucracy and the processes of politics. He even learned to enjoy them, and occasionally to laugh at them.

He and the state directors were busy men in 1924. The Rehabilitation Act was scheduled to expire that year unless Congress could be persuaded to renew it. It was a Presidential election year, with President Coolidge to face the electorate for the first time as a Presidential candidate. Unlike present-day Congressional schedules, the Congress would adjourn in June and would not be in session until the new Congress convened in December.

The Congress extended the Federal law but not without some struggles and some curious legislative mishaps.

Following House passage of the bill, the Senate was engaged in a debate on the bill when an argument arose over how long the program should be continued. The bill before the Senate called for extending the program for another four years. A few Senators, notably Senator King of Utah, were insisting that the law should be extended for only two years. In charge of the bill and urging a four-year extension was Simeon D. Fess, the former Ohio Congressman who had championed the bill in 1920 and who now was a United States Senator. He invited Senator King to come forward and mark the bill in the way Senator King wished it to read. Senator King marked the bill—but he did not take the time to see what his handiwork had produced. He had changed the bill in such a way that it provided for an extension of six years—and the bill passed the Senate in that form.

The confusion was not ended. When the Senate-House conferees met to adjust the differences between the two bills, they were in agreement that the program should be extended for three years—but again a language error was committed, with the result that the bill as finally reported from conference, and enacted, authorized $1 million annually for six years.

With so many faux pas in its legislative history, the new law ended up under review by the U. S. Comptroller, who ruled that it was the intent of Congress to provide a six-year extension of the Act. So the program had a new lease on life until 1930.

It was natural, and in this case necessary, that the state directors of vocational rehabilitation should form an organization to protect and advance their interests. It came into being first in 1924 as the National Civilian Rehabilitation Conference with W. F. Faulkes as Chairman. From that beginning group, the organization evolved into the National Rehabilitation Association in 1927, with Marlow Perrin, state director of the Ohio program, as President. The meeting that year gave much time to the question of membership and who would be accepted as full-fledged members. Having so recently "dis-affiliated" from the National Society for Vocational Education, and with much evidence that the Federal-state program probably would stand or fall on their own efforts, many of the state directors felt that full membership should be limited to personnel of the public program. Others felt the new organization needed the participation and help of many other people. Ira W. Kirby of the California vocational rehabilitation program was one of these in the minority. Dr. Henry H. Kessler and his mentor from the war days, Dr. Fred Albee, urged the group to open membership to all persons in rehabilitation work. But they did not prevail and the early NRA functioned entirely under the control of the Federal-state personnel.

Many of the emerging programs and organizations already were seeking ways to fuse together the professions and the institutionalized systems in public and private life, to concentrate a variety of skills upon the specialized problems of the disabled. Henry Edward Abt, Director of Information of the International Society for Crippled Children made such a plea in 1924: ". . . The needs of crippled children are so varied as to place demands on many diversified fields of social activity. There is a great army of pediatricians, orthopedists, and general physicians to whom the crippled child is but one of a great mass of individuals requiring physical and constitutional remedy . . . The physically handicapped form a distinct educational problem. Similarly, those who aim to relieve destitution are constantly confronted with the necessity of aiding these cases. To those who provide vocational guidance and to those who operate industries, cripples have always been a problem.

"The great danger in these activities is that the ultimate solution will become a mirage to each crippled individual. Those who would aim to provide remedy without cooperating with educators to make available school facilities, place the child in the position of the prospector who has discovered gold, but has no means of transporting it to metropolitan markets. Those who would educate without cooperating with others who would relieve hunger, are equally culpable. Educational facilities which do not cooperate with the agencies which render vocational assistance are quite ineffective."

As interest grew in the problems of disabled children and adults, a few physicians were attracted to the idea of using some of the physical therapy methods to alleviate and change chronic conditions. They were a rare and often lonely breed at that time but a few were convinced that the use of physical agents, if researched, expanded and more broadly used, could lead to significant advances in overcoming a great variety of disabling conditions.

One of these was Dr. John Stanley Coulter who not only pioneered in physical medicine in the United States but in 1926 became Assistant Professor of Physical Therapy on the faculty of Northwestern University Medical School, becoming thereby one of the earliest physicians to initiate such a program in a university setting.

This was a period when the public and voluntary programs for the disabled could and did join in some of the prosperity. Fund-raising was easier, legislators more willing to spend. Post-war unemployment fears had subsided, jobs were plentiful in most places and there was money for many things. There was money for thousands of college boys to wear raccoon coats, money for their "flapper" girl friends to wear scandalously short skirts and twirl their beads, money for bathtub gin and *College Humor.* There was enough money to make John Held rich and famous with his drawings of the kids and enough to encourage Henry Ford to launch his first Model A.

Without much money, Charles Lindbergh flew his "Spirit of St. Louis" nonstop from New York to Paris in 1927. Many people said this meant that one of these days, a person would be able to fly all the way from the United States to Europe, whenever he wanted to. But a lot of people disagreed, insisting that if the Lord had meant for men to fly, He would have made them with wings. Some of the less religious just snickered and said that flying was for the birds.

As the 1928 Presidential election neared, Republican party leaders increasingly pressed President Coolidge for an answer: Would he be a candidate for re-election? In his own good time, President Coolidge gave them an answer in his characteristic fashion: "I do not choose to run."

And so the party turned to Herbert Clark Hoover to carry the party colors against the powerful and experienced Democratic candidate, Governor Alfred E. Smith of New York.

Hoover was the well-to-do but not wealthy man who had elected to give much of his life to public service and to give up a fortune in the process.

He had gotten involved back in the years of the Boxer Rebellion in China, where he had gone as head of an engineering firm, and where he found himself unofficially responsible for organizing the American compound in Tientsin when it was under attack. There had followed his massive task of relief work in Europe in World War I, which had begun in 1914—again in a time when he was there at the head of his large and prosperous engineering firm. With the outbreak of the war in Europe, thousands of Americans stranded there presented an emergency problem for the United States. When the American Consul called on a Monday morning to ask Hoover to take on the task of repatriating them, he accepted—and said much later: ". . . On this Monday, my engineering career was over. I was on the slippery road of public life."

His wartime service, as director of the Commission for Relief in Belgium and as President Wilson's appointee as head of the U. S. Food Administration in 1917—in which he had exercised great power over prices, production and distribution—made him fairly well known to the voters, who had adopted the term "Hooverize" to describe saving or doing without many items that were scarce in wartime.

The Democratic nominee, Governor Smith, entered the campaign with political experience and skills which probably were unmatched at the time. At least in the East, he was considered to be closer to the "common man," with his bluff oratory and his direct approach to precinct politics, than his opponent. But outside the Eastern cities, there were many questions, for Smith was a Roman Catholic, he bore the label of Tammany Hall, and he favored the repeal of Prohibition. He made many speeches; Hoover made only seven.

When the votes were counted and the electoral ballots tallied, Hoover had carried forty of the forty-eight states; he received 444 electoral vote to 87 for Smith.

In his first year of the Presidency, Mr. Hoover organized a national conference on the health and protection of children. He raised $500,000 privately to cover the costs of the conference, which was attended by more than 1,200 delegates.

In opening the conference, President Hoover said, in

part: "Our problem falls in three groups: first, the protection and stimulation of the normal child; second, aid to the physically defective and handicapped child; third, the problem of the delinquent child." He cited statistics indicating that, of 45 million children, 1 million had defective speech, 1 million had weak or damaged hearts, 450,000 were mentally retarded, 382,000 were afflicted with tuberculosis, 342,000 had impaired hearing, 18,000 were totally deaf, 300,000 were otherwise crippled, and 64,000 were partially or totally blind.

He and Dr. Ray Lyman Wilbur and the conferees developed from the conference a "children's charter" which set forth nineteen national goals for children, one of which stated: "For every child who is blind, deaf, crippled, or otherwise physically handicapped, and for the child who is mentally handicapped, such measures as will early discover and diagnose his handicap, provide care and treatment, and so train him that he may become an asset to society rather than a liability. Expenses of these services should be borne publicly where they cannot be privately met."

By this time many of the early programs had their "feet on the ground" and were struggling with the more mundane problems of successful operation and slow growth. In 1928, the Institute for the Crippled and Disabled celebrated its tenth anniversary, with world heavyweight champion Gene Tunney telling the anniversary dinner guests: "I personally believe that every boy and girl in this Institute has shown more courage in one day than I have been called upon to show in my whole career as a boxer."

In the same year, the state rehabilitation program in Virginia acquired a new director. Richard N. Anderson, former superintendent of public schools in Russell County, took over a rehabilitation program with a budget of $21,342. There scarcely was any way for him to foresee that, by the time he retired in 1961, he would be dealing with many millions of dollars and that the Virginia program by 1970 would be spending around $20,000,000

In Wisconsin, the Curative Workshop of Milwaukee named Miss Marjorie Taylor as its new executive in 1928. From her post as director of occupational therapy training at Milwaukee-Downer College, Miss Taylor first assumed the directorship of the workshop on a part-time basis and then went on to become a nationally known figure in the development of advance programs for the disabled through comprehensive workshop services.

The wide-ranging interests of Jeremiah Milbank in medical research and rehabilitation took another turn in 1928. After many conversations with the leading researchers of the day, he organized and financed an International Committee for the Study of Infantile Paralysis, probably the earliest large-scale effort to make an organized attack on the enigmatic disease which was killing and disabling thousands of children every year. The thirteen Committee members, each an eminent scientist, guided the work, most of it done through support of forty-five researchers in universities conducting laboratory and other studies on various phases of the project.

The results of the undertaking, published at the conclusion of the Committee's work in 1932 in the book, *Poliomyelitis* by the Williams and Wilkins Company of Baltimore, provided one of the first comprehensive documentations on the total characteristics of polio. The Committee did not produce an answer to the polio problem but one of the participating researchers, Dr. A. B. Sabin, would live to do just that.

In most places in the late Twenties, the rehabilitation effort was moving steadily ahead in a national economy where confidence was the watchword, boom talk was the

favorite conversation and fortunes were being made overnight.

Few were prepared for the catastrophe which descended upon the country with the stock market crash of
1929. The crash was more than the loss of personal fortunes. It was a paralyzing blow to the companies whose
money was represented by all those shares of stock—money
for operations and expansion, money which now disappeared in worthless pieces of paper stock.

Companies of all kinds, large and small, in all sorts
of industrial and commercial lines, folded. With them went
hundreds of thousands of jobs.

It was a nightmare for most of the country. And if you
were trying to raise money to train disabled people, if you
were trying to place them in jobs where every opening had
a hundred able-bodied applicants, you could be excused if
you gave up.

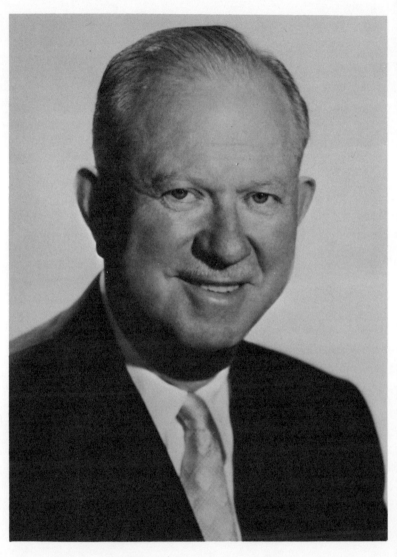

HENRY H. KESSLER, M.D.

Chapter IV

SURVIVAL

———◆•••◆———

OUT OF THE SHOCKS and tremors of the 1929 crash and the onset of the Great Depression came a period when the dominant words in government and many other places were caution and restraint. There could be no resumption of growth or even normalcy until the waves of panic subsided, the loss of hope was restored.

From somewhere there must come the money and methods to put several million people back to work, to revive business, to begin a new flow of taxes into the treasury, to demonstrate with jobs that the people and the nation did indeed have a future.

One of the remarkable things about the period was that most of the rehabilitation programs, public and private, were able to survive. The people who had given so much of themselves in a commitment to the disabled of the nation were not the kind to give up easily. Many of the people who had contributed their personal funds, large and small, to make these beginnings suddenly had no money to give but their moral support, and their confidence in the face of this new calamity helped sustain many organizations that otherwise would have disappeared.

The public program came through another crucial test in 1930 when the Congress, despite the critical financial situation, extended the Federal-state rehabilitation law again and President Hoover signed the new statute on June 9. The same amount of annual grant funds for the states, $1 million, was continued for another three years.

That year one of the creative planners of the public program, Terry Foster of the Federal staff, prepared one of the early basic documents on the nature of vocational rehabilitation and the functions of the counselor. He foresaw a broadening role for the program in the coming years. In the continuing effort to define the nature of rehabilitation counseling and the role of the counselor (who was called an "agent" at that time) he made one thing clear: "The rehabilitation agent is a professional worker . . ."

In Peoria, Illinois the city fathers could take time in 1930 to consider the problems of blind people and pass the Nation's first city ordinance governing observance of the white cane used by the blind.

And in 1930, despite the financial panics, Jeremiah Milbank made one of his largest contributions to begin building a new Institute for the Crippled and Disabled, probably the first designed specifically to serve as a comprehensive rehabilitation center.

In 1931 the growing vocational rehabilitation program in Pennsylvania acquired a new state director, Mark M. Walter—and for the future of rehabilitation in Pennsylvania and throughout the nation, it was a very fortunate appointment.

The American Occupational Therapy Association, after several years of concentrated work on the improvement of its educational standards, issued its first registry of professionally trained occupational therapists—a list which totalled just 318.

The nation's health authorities, particularly in public health, faced their share of worries. The senior ones could recall the days before the turn of the century and for some time after, when epidemics were frequent and uncontrollable. But in their lifetimes they had seen the conquest and control of most of these diseases, the elevation of health protection on such a dramatic scale that they saw a depression as a potential reversion to mass outbreaks of diseases they knew how to control.

It had been, indeed, an impressive set of victories, as noted many years later by Samuel Eliot Morison in his *The Oxford History of the American People:* "In the first third of the century, infant mortality in the United States declined by two-thirds, and life expectancy increased from 49 to 59 years. The death rate for tuberculosis dropped from 180 to 49 per 100,000, for typhoid from 36 to two, for diphtheria from 43 to two, for measles from 12 to one, for pneumonia from 158 to 50 . . . yellow fever and smallpox were practically wiped out and the war on malaria, pellagra, hookworm, and similar diseases was brilliantly successful."

But these gains, like others, would not sustain themselves. For them to be held and advanced, the country must be solvent, business must be encouraged and aided to begin again, and the wheels of both industry and normal living must start turning again.

The election of Franklin D. Roosevelt in 1932 as the thirty-second President was the beginning, not only of the longest White House tenure of any President, but of thrashing about in Washington, "fire-side chats" to reach the people by radio, and the launching of dozens of new governmental programs. There were drastic measures, such as the "bank holiday" which began on the day of Roosevelt's inauguration in 1933 and closed every bank in the country, many of them never to open again. In one of the fastest

Constitutional amendments to be approved by the people, the Prohibition law was ended that year. There followed the alphabet agencies of FERA (Federal Emergency Relief Administration), the WPA (Works Progress Administration), the PWA (Public Works Administration), and a new form of the NRA (the National Recovery Administration).

Again the United States had a President who had some first-hand knowledge of disability. Franklin D. Roosevelt had been a victim of polio in 1921 and would be a polio paraplegic for the rest of his life. In his determination to remain active and to master his disability, he did many things, including establishing a foundation which created the famed center at Warm Springs, Georgia.

While the machinery of the New Deal was being assembled, many of the future leaders in rehabilitation were struggling with the simple tasks of making a living. One of these was a young physician named Dr. Miland E. Knapp who completed a surgical residency at Minneapolis General Hospital in 1933 and was facing a situation familiar to hundreds of young physicians finishing training in those years. He found himself named chief of the Department of Physical Therapy at the hospital because he had shown particular interest in treatment and restoration of function in fractures. Since he knew little about the field, he spent two weeks at Michael Rees Hospital in Chicago with Dr. Charles Molander and accompanied Dr. John S. Coulter on medical rounds at several Chicago hospitals.

When he returned to Minneapolis and entered general practice, he had plenty of free time to spend in the Department of Physical Therapy at Minneapolis General. As he recounted many years later, in the first six months of his practice he never had a gross income which exceeded fifty dollars a month. His next and eventful step is described by Dr. Knapp this way: "In spite of the total lack of interest in my surgical training, I found that many of the doctors were asking me questions about physical therapy and it seemed that this field could be developed. Therefore, after nine months of general practice I decided to go into this new field as a specialty before I built up enough medical practice to worry about dropping it. Therefore, I rented an office in the Medical Arts building and put my name on the door with the notation, 'Practice Limited to Physical Therapy.'

"Then I starved for three years."

For the public program, it was time to begin work again on that perennial problem—getting the Federal law extended again. John Kratz and his colleagues were not people to wait upon the course of events. He had worked before with Dr. John J. Lee, Chairman of the legislative committee of the National Rehabilitation Association in extending the Act and now, in the midst of endless changes of policies and programs in Washington, the task must be faced all over again.

But there was a preliminary project—a visit to President Roosevelt's key man in the White House, Harry Hopkins, to propose what probably was the first specific plan to rehabilitate into employment disabled people from the welfare rolls. Kratz asked for a special appropriation of some $70,000 monthly for two years (1934 and 1935) to be used only to provide vocational rehabilitation services to public assistance cases. This found favor with Hopkins and with the President, and the funds were furnished a little later by transfer from the Federal Emergency Relief Administration.

The next step was aimed at the basic problem of the temporary nature of the Federal law. The approach taken this time by Kratz and his associates was different. They were convinced that the new Social Security bill, then in the early stages of development, would pass. They would "ride" the bill by getting a provision included to give permanent authorization for continuation of the Vocational Rehabilitation Act and its programs.

Mr. Kratz, now teamed with Mark Walter of Pennsylvania in the program's legislative missions, described in later years their approach: ". . . in his first year in office (President Roosevelt) appointed a commission to study and make recommendations on the nation's need for a program of Social Security. A friend of mine (Jay Howenstine), the Executive Secretary of the National Society for Crippled Children, advised me that he had learned what might be the trend of thinking of this commission and the probable types of service they would include in their legislative recommendations. I concluded that I had better see for myself what might be in the offing for rehabilitation. I got in touch with my good friend Bill Faulkes, Chief of Vocational Rehabilitation for Wisconsin. He knew very well the Executive Secretary of the President's commission and took me to see him. We tried to get an invitation to appear before the commission but at that time they had adjourned their hearing and were in the process of preparing their report. However, we did our best to convince the secretary that vocational rehabilitation was definitely a part of any plan for Social Security. We also indicated the desirability of inclusion in the commission's report of recommendations of some form of legislation putting our program on a permanent basis.

"When the commission report was published it did contain a short section on vocational rehabilitation, indicating its place in a security program, but made no recommendations as to legislation. We had gained a point but we felt we should attempt some further means of getting a legislative provision for the permanency of our program. We reasoned that on the basis of the commission's recommendations, the Congress would pass social security legislation, and if rehabilitation were to be included in the proposed bill, it would remain in the bill as finally passed. It appeared obvious, therefore, that we would have to go directly to the Congress, but before doing so we would have to obtain backing of someone on the President's commission.

"We arranged for a committee to call on Frances Perkins, Secretary of Labor, and top government members of the Security Commission. This committee consisted of Dr. R. M. Little, Director of Vocational Rehabilitation, New York State, M. M. Walter, Chairman of the Legislative Committee of the National Rehabilitation Association, and myself representing the Federal office. Dr. Little knew Miss Perkins when she was Secretary of Labor for New York State, and arranged an appointment for us with her deputy, Mr. Arthur Altmeyer, who later became the Chairman of the Social Security Board when it was established under the Social Security Act of 1935.

"The proposal for legislation which we presented to Mr. Altmeyer, who was acting for Miss Perkins, was that a provision be included in the then pending social security bill which would do the following: (1) make a permanent authorization of Federal appropriations for rehabilitation grants to the states; and (2) increase the current authorization of appropriations from $1 million to $2 million per annum.

"The result of this conference with Altmeyer was that the President's commission raised no objection to our proposed amendment to their social security bill. This was a great gain for us, but the big job that lay ahead was that of getting a Congressional sponsor for our proposal and the approval of the Ways and Means Committee of the House which was considering the social security bill. In this respect we were very fortunate. Mr. Dan Reed, a Congressman from New York State, who at this time was a ranking Republican of the House (Ways and Means) Committee, was an old friend. I had known and worked with him when we were pushing our rehabilitation legislation in the House in 1924. At that time he was chairman of the House Committee on Education which was handling our rehabilitation bill. Consequently he was familiar with our program and friendly to me and Mark Walter. No difficulty was encountered in securing his agreement to sponsor our proposed amendment to the social security bill and at the opportune time he proposed the amendment and the Ways and Means Committee accepted it.

"Dr. R. M. Little appeared before the Committee in support of the amendment as did Mark Walter, representing the NRA. Later on I appeared for the proposal when the bill was being considered in the Senate. When the bill passed the House it carried our amendment, as it did also in the Senate. This was in 1935, and our troubles were over with respect to the need for further extensions of our basic act."

At the time, this achievement meant something important to a relative handful of people—the 150 or so people who constituted the entire Federal-state program.

To most other people, the Social Security Act meant a new national insurance system to provide incomes for the retired. But it was more than that. There would be protection for those laid off from work, through a new system of unemployment benefits; a nationwide public employment service to help find jobs for those out of work and to help employers find workers; and a beginning for a national welfare system in which the Federal government would share the costs with the state for various categories of poor people.

While Washington was seething with the controversies that swirled round the New Deal programs, the Institute for the Crippled and Disabled in New York quietly made a major change in its rehabilitation program for the disabled. It installed, as part of its institutional program a medical service component, directed by Dr. George D. Deaver, so that the Institute no longer would have to rely on the willingness and capabilities of city hospitals and clinics for their disabled people. It was the beginning of a highly creative program of physical restoration which strongly reinforced the social and vocational elements of the Institute's program.

It also was the year when Dr. Henry Kessler published one of his many major contributions to the rehabilitation literature, this one a book *The Crippled and the Disabled* which soon became a textbook in the teaching of rehabilitation personnel in the United States. It came at a valuable time. Although the rehabilitation "movement" had continued to develop into the Thirties, the concept of a comprehensive medical-social-psychological-vocational type of approach to the difficult problems of the chronically disabled had not materialized in many places.

Beginnings had been made with such public health problems as tuberculosis (notably through the Trudeau Society and the work of the Altro Workshop), but for most other chronic conditions, the idea of medical rehabilitation had not yet evolved. In his 1935 book, Dr. Kessler observed: "It is very difficult to place chronic invalids in appropriate institutions. They are usually found in alms houses which have no facilities for their care. Some hospitals refuse them admission because they can retain them for only a short period of time and have no place to which to discharge them. Homes for the aged often reject them because they are not equipped to care for them. The problem of the chronic invalid therefore is most acute."

Such a mild statement of a national problem was not forthcoming from Dr. Kessler very often. His experience as a surgeon had shown him the intense personal agonies, the human dislocations and the social consequences of neglecting the disabled. Out of his association with Dr. Fred Albee in World War I he had seen a vision of what could be accomplished if the necessary skills, money and facilities were concentrated on the solution of a handicapped person's problems.

His concern with the victims of industrial accidents and the widespread defects in workmen's compensation began early in his professional life and continued throughout his career. He endeavored to provide some measure of protection and restoration through his work on the original New Jersey vocational rehabilitation law, through his work with the Congress in the enactment and succeeding amendments to the National Rehabilitation Act, and through countless meetings and proceedings on the relationship between workmen's compensation and the disabled people it was designed to protect and help. He had gone beyond the clinical problems and studied carefully the technical methods of rating systems for disability claims under workmen's compensation, and in 1931 published the first American text on the subject, *Accidental Injuries.*

He was a strong advocate of bringing rehabilitation programs, public and private, closer together, both in their professional lives and in their planning for meeting national needs. He was one of the very few doctors who displayed a sustained interest in the early development of the National Rehabilitation Association. He alternately begged and besieged his fellow orthopedic surgeons in an effort to gain widespread professional interest and responsibility for going beyond the immediate requirement of good surgery and seeing the patient through to a renewed and useful place in life.

As an orthopedist, he had a natural interest in amputee problems and in the associated problems of amputation surgery and the preparation of the stump, in proper fitting and training, and in the research effort required to constantly improve artificial limbs.

But beyond his extensive professional schedule, he continued to inveigh against the shortcomings and inequities of most state workmen's compensation systems. He argued vigorously against lump-sum settlements and against laws which permitted litigation to extend for so long that there was little or no hope of eventual rehabilitation of the disabled person the law was supposed to help. Years later, it was obvious that his ardor for the subject had not cooled. Writing in *Rehabilitation Literature* in 1965, he recalled the early days in New Jersey in these words:

"As all patients (in the New Jersey Rehabilitation Commission program) were injured workers, complete control over the program of medical care was in the hands of the insurance companies. Unfortunately, in spite of the importunings of Dr. Albee and Colonel Bryant, the companies failed to cooperate. Anxious to dispose of their cases with financial settlements, they saw no moral or legal responsibility to go beyond the extremely limited provisions for medical benefit in the Workmen's Compensation Act. Here was a golden opportunity to do for disabled workers what the government was doing for the war wounded, but a narrow, immediate, parochial, economic interpretation deprived the public of a greater economic and social opportunity. As Workmen's Compensation has continued to drift during the past fifty years from a hopeful blessing for all injured workers to a gambling arena and bazaar for hungry litigants, rehabilitation has been stomped, strangled, and emasculated by the demon of indemnity."

What bothered Dr. Kessler in 1935 and in all those succeeding years has not been resolved yet. As long as conditions are created and sustained, in workmen's compensation or any other program, which make it more profitable to neglect the disabled than to restore them to activity and productivity, the problem will remain unresolved.

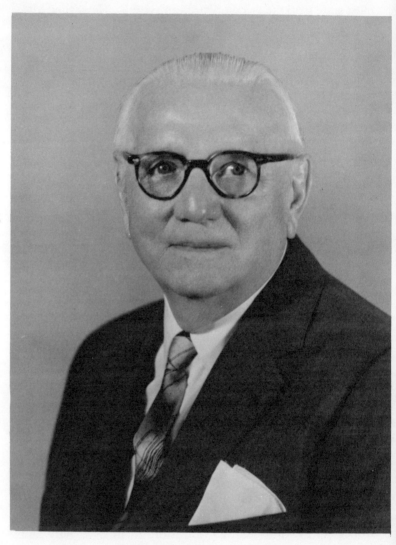

FRANK H. KRUSEN, M.D.

CHAPTER V

RENEWAL

————◆◆◆◆————

GETTING THE NATION'S economic train back on the track in the Thirties was a slow and discouraging task but the emergency measures began to show results. The apple-sellers began to disappear from street corners and many of the deflated stocks began to come to life in a stock market newly regulated under a Securities Exchange Commission.

The public rehabilitation program could report a total of 9,422 handicapped people rehabilitated into employment in 1935, an excellent growth in services over the 523 restored back in 1921. Most of the voluntary groups were recovering and moving ahead again, with Goodwill Industries local units operating in 64 communities by the late 1930's.

In Washington, a young Congressman from West Virginia, Jennings Randolph, sponsored a bill with Senator Sheppard to help blind people find self-employment. The bill called for the Federal government to give preference to blind persons in establishing and operating vending stands in Federal buildings. Not everyone was convinced that blind persons could handle such a job, entailing the ordering, stocking and inventorying of a variety of merchandise, the hiring of help, the recordkeeping, the daily work with the public. But Jennings Randolph and most of his colleagues, in and out of government, were convinced they could. When the bill passed in 1936, it was the beginning of one of the Federal government's most successful efforts for handicapped people, the Randolph-Sheppard Vending Stand Program for the Blind, which not only was a success in Federal buildings but paved the way for most states to make similar arrangements in state-owned buildings.

Two years later the Congress again acted on behalf of the nation's blind citizens, passing the Wagner-O'Day Act which made provision for the government to regularly buy various of its supply items from workshops for the blind, so that a source of contract work for the blind employees was assured.

For most people, there were increasing signs of recovery from the long depression. Wages were still low but there were more jobs. College enrollments were on the increase again. Bennie Goodman and his orchestra were playing to packed audiences on the Steel Pier in Atlantic City. *Gone with the Wind,* which had been a phenomenal best-seller, earned the 1937 Pulitzer Prize for author Margaret Mitchell.

As part of the metamorphosis of the Crippled Children's organization, the International Society for the Welfare of Cripples came into being in 1938. The Ohio Society for Crippled Children, formed in 1919, had attracted the interest of people in other states and, by 1921, it became the National Society for Crippled Children, with six state organizations affiliated. The following year the organization broadened its sights to become the International Society for Crippled Children.

However, in 1938, a division occurred between the domestic and international aims of the organization and the U. S. group became once again the National Society for

Crippled Children. In the process, the International Society for the Welfare of Cripples was born, providing a continuing and growing forum for cooperation between numerous countries, notably Canada, and marking the beginning of the foremost international organization concerned with disabled people.

The famed Mayo Clinic in Rochester, Minnesota added a new man and a new section in 1935 which would become the springboard for one of the nation's outstanding figures in rehabilitation. Dr. Frank H. Krusen, who in 1929 had established a department of physical medicine at Temple University, joined the Mayo Clinic to organize and direct their first section devoted to the use of physical agents in the treatment of disease, injury and disabling conditions. The following year there was established at the Mayo Graduate School of Medicine the first three-year fellowships in physical medicine, setting the stage for later organized training programs for physicians and for the day when they would be recognized through a specialty board of their own. The physical therapy school was growing and providing some of the best-trained therapists of the day.

When the American Academy of Physical Medicine was first organized in 1936, Dr. Krusen was elected President, beginning a long series of high professional offices and honors.

Dr. Krusen had begun early to contribute to the literature for his field both in research and professional teaching. His first small book was *Physical Therapy in Arthritis,* published in 1937. Four years later he published his basic and massive text, *Physical Medicine,* which became the definitive work in the field.

The long-range effects of Dr. Krusen's trail-blazing at Mayo on the future of the field were immense. It would be largely Dr. Krusen's graduates from his educational program of the late Thirties and the early Forties who would become the clinicians, the researchers, the teachers and the torch-bearers for the growth period that lay ahead.

In 1940 Sister Elizabeth Kenney arrived in Minneapolis to begin at the University of Minnesota and the Minneapolis General Hospital her controversial new methods of treatment for poliomyelitis patients. Even while she and her techniques were being investigated, there was a prompt demand for training more personnel to use the Kenney method, and courses were started, with the aid of the National Foundation for Infantile Paralysis.

There was no one to foresee how the future of the Kenney work and the career of Dr. Krusen would one day come together in a mammoth effort to save one of America's finest rehabilitation institutions.

The Federal government at that time was engaged in its periodic ritual of reorganizing. This one was of more than passing interest to the rehabilitation field. Since its beginning, the vocational rehabilitation organization had been largely submerged in the bureaucracy as far as authority and visibility were concerned. In 1939 the Federal Security Agency (forerunner of the Department of Health, Education and Welfare) was created, bringing together in one Federal agency the programs in Social Security, education, welfare, the Public Health Service and its programs (which had been in the U. S. Treasury Department) and certain others.

The reorganization established an Office of Vocational Rehabilitation as a new and separate agency, reporting directly to the Administrator of the Federal Security Agency, Paul McNutt. Named to head the new OVR was Michael J. Shortley, with Mr. Kratz as deputy.

Now the rehabilitation agency would be better able to plan its program, develop its budget and participate in the larger framework of policy making. Now there would be the administrative climate for leadership and growth.

As the depression began to recede, there were other problems to be faced. The "dust bowl" years were upon much of the southwest and the "Okies" and others were leaving the barren remains of their farms for what they hoped would be a new chance in California. Their agonies and their migration, which came alive in *The Grapes of Wrath,* launched John Steinbeck as a foremost figure in American literature.

Spencer Tracy set a record by winning two Motion Picture Academy Oscars in a row, for his "Captains Courageous" in 1937 and "Boys Town" in 1938.

In New York in 1939, a vast amount of publicity was focused on the opening of the New York World's Fair. Not far away, at Columbia University, there was much less publicity on the fact that scientists there had, for the first time, split the uranium atom.

Across the Atlantic, the machinery of war was being oiled again in Germany. Adolf Hitler and his Brown Shirts had carried out unsuccessful putsches before but now they *were* Germany and it only remained to see how far their shouts for "lebensraum" would be heard. Italy allied itself with the new German power to the north. On September 7, 1940, Japan signed a ten-year pact with the Axis powers, which had the effect of assuring that the German-Italian drive could proceed without interruption in Europe, while the Japanese could pursue their plans in Asia and the Pacific. Three weeks later Japan attacked French Indo-China.

Slowly, steadily the inevitability of war for the United States became clearer. President Roosevelt and the Congress were willing to help the British and French defenses, although issues like "Lend-Lease" were bitterly argued in the Congress. Even more strenuous was the debate over instituting a draft. The draft bill passed in 1940 but for one year only, and thousands of draftees marched off to the induction stations to the song, "I'll Be Back in a Year, Little Darling"—but few of them were. When renewal of the draft law came before the Congress in 1941, the debate dragged on into September. It finally carried—by one vote in the House.

On December 7, 1941 the need for a draft became quite clear. The Japanese attack on Pearl Harbor in Hawaii (and on the Philippines, Midway and Wake Islands and Guam) eliminated any vestige of hope for peace. The United States was at war again, this time on a truly world scale.

And once again, the United States was unprepared for war and the aftermath of war.

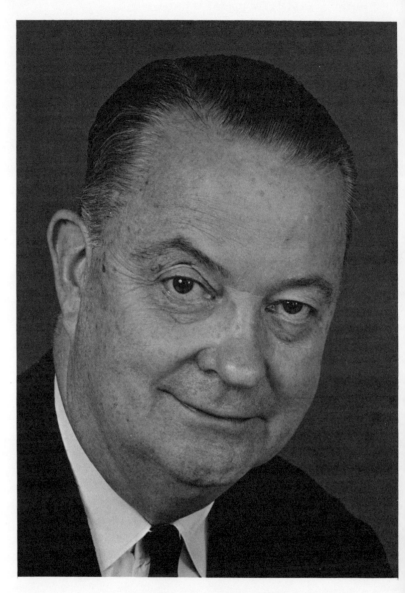

HOWARD A. RUSK, M.D.

CHAPTER VI

THE FRUITS OF TRAGEDY

THE FOUR-YEAR RECORD of Hitler's march through Europe and North Africa, the series of Japanese forays in China, Burma and Indo-China, had not been sufficient to induce the United States to prepare for war.

In 1940 the entire U. S. Armed Forces totalled less than half a million men. (By the end of the war, they would total nearly fourteen million men.)

In 1940 the Army Air Corps consisted of slightly over 51,000 officers and men who had for combat use about 2,800 aircraft, all of which were outdated and lacked the firepower and performance characteristics of the German and Japanese planes.

In general, the Navy was in a comparable situation with respect to naval craft, particularly following the Japanese attack upon Pearl Harbor and the destruction of naval vessels there.

The Army's situation was similar, with largely outmoded combat equipment, only limited development of modern tanks and armored vehicles, and a critical shortage of the many types of vehicles needed for logistical support. Army draftees entering service in the early days of the draft were given musty uniforms and worn equipment left over from World War I.

Setting the draft in motion in the winter of 1940–1941 probably was a decisive factor in securing some degree of preparation for the United States. In addition to the thousands of young men added to augment the small regular forces, the draft launched all sorts of preparatory measures: contracts were let to begin building the new military bases required to accommodate the men, other contracts were let to procure uniforms, more modern rifles and other equipment, medical supplies and dozens of other essentials for maintaining an increased military force; the command organizations of the Army, Navy, Air Force and Marine Corps were changed, to accommodate themselves to an expansion in the size of troop strength; and new provisions were made for transporting, on a large scale, vast numbers of men and matériel.

Compared with previous wars, the United States was somewhat better prepared to deal with the sick, the injured and the disabled, but not much. Certainly the armed forces did not, and could not, have on standby the type and volume of hospitals and other care facilities, both at home and abroad, that would be needed—not after those lean years of the Thirties.

There were some pluses in the picture in terms of capacity to provide rehabilitation programs for disabled veterans. This was largely due to two factors—the active role played by major veterans organizations such as the American Legion, the Disabled American Veterans and the Veterans of Foreign Wars, and the existence and growing capabilities of the Federal-state vocational rehabilitation program.

One result of this was to project a controversy in government over placing the responsibility for the vocational rehabilitation of returning veterans. A strenuous effort was made by White House advisors and others to assign to the Office of Vocational Rehabilitation and its cooperating state agencies the responsibility for carrying out an expanded program to rehabilitate returning disabled veterans. This move was hotly contested, not only by the Veterans Administration but even more effectively by the veterans organizations, following their traditional policy of seeking separate programs of benefits for veterans.

The Veterans Administration at that time was not in a strong position to decide such an issue. The agency had been in trouble of one sort or another most of the time since it was created to meet the needs of World War I veterans. It had suffered from a scandal during the Harding Administration and in 1933 the old Veterans Bureau was reorganized as the Veterans Administration. For a variety of reasons, including extremely limited appropriations during the depression years of the Thirties, the Veterans Administration was at least as unprepared for a world war as the rest of the government. It had, however, one vast advantage over the situation following World War I: it had a system of hospitals, however good or bad, which meant a base to build upon. It also had the advantage, as did the Congress of having learned from World War I a lot of things not to do.

For a while, though, it appeared that these earlier mistakes would not be remembered or heeded. The proposals to provide, through the Office of Vocational Rehabilitation, an expanded program of vocational rehabilitation for both veterans and non-veterans, were an example. Bills were introduced to this effect by several Senators and Congressmen, including Senator Robert La Follette and Congressman Graham Barden, who were to figure strongly in civilian rehabilitation legislation. But predictably, the result was a series of hearings, new bills, meetings and a relative stalemate.

By March, 1943 a bill was agreed to which vested in the Veterans Administration the responsibility for providing vocational rehabilitation services to disabled veterans and it was signed by President Roosevelt on March 24 as Public Law 16, 78th Congress.

More than a year later, the broader program of benefits for all veterans, the "GI bill" (Public Law 346, 78th Congress) was enacted into law. Thus the disabled veteran of World War II had benefits under two laws—a general educational program for veterans and a special program for disabled veterans.

With the earlier decision to proceed with separate legislation for veterans, it became necessary to begin work on revisions in the Federal law for the civilian vocational rehabilitation program. Obviously the program would have to be geared up to a broader job in helping to meet wartime manpower needs. Operationally, this was readily understood and agreed to in government circles; provisions were made to protect most rehabilitation counselors from the draft, so the agencies could continue and expand their work, and special arrangements were made to automatically refer to the state rehabilitation agencies the thousands of young men turned down in the draft for physical defects. The latter arrangement sounded good but, according to many of the state directors at the time and later, served more to clog up the paperwork system than to increase the numbers of disabled people rehabilitated for military or industrial jobs.

Getting the legislative wheels turning to broaden the Act was done less by government policy decision than by the initiative and persistence of John Kratz and Mark Walter and others. Something had to be done to permit the rehabilitation agencies to have physical defects removed or modified, to assume the costs of living for disabled clients while they were in training, to serve some of the mentally handicapped who had prospects of responding to proper measures and becoming employable, and to change the Federal-state financing system to offer a greater inducement to the states to expand and improve their programs. The state agencies were feeling the pressures from many directions as war plants, offices, service companies and others were pleading for employees in many places, as the draft steadily drained off their workers.

Mr. Kratz and Mr. Walter (himself a lawyer) were able to get a bill drafted by the legal counsel of the Social Security Administration and to begin searching for someone on "The Hill" to sponsor it. Mr. Kratz described their odyssey this way:

"When the draft of the bill was completed, we encountered some difficulty in securing a House sponsor . . . The Committee (on Education and Labor) was chaired by an elderly representative from Indiana, a Dr. Larrabee. He had not had a meeting of his Committee in eighteen months. We made some investigation of possible sponsors high on the Committee's roster and learned that Graham A. Barden of North Carolina was a competent and reliable legislator and might be interested. Mr. Walter and his legislative committee of the NRA secured an appointment with the chairman of the Committee, and I accompanied them. The chairman received us standing in his outer office. We advised him of our need for a sponsor, and indirectly suggested Mr. Barden. As direct as we had been indirect, the chairman informed us that he did not appreciate being told how to run his Committee but would consider the matter. We then went to Mr. Barden and told him what we had done. He was inclined to sponsor our bill but said he would consult the chairman. Shortly thereafter we learned that Barden had been assigned the chairmanship of a subcommittee to handle our bill and conduct hearings on it . . . Mr. Barden took over and introduced our bill. In addition, in a short time, the chairman retired and Mr. Barden succeeded him as chairman of the whole Committee. This put the Barden bill in excellent position for hearings . . . Mark had his NRA group behind him, which organization he represented, and I had the 'go' sign from our Social Security Assistant Administrator, Watson Miller. Miller told me it was my responsibility to carry the legislative ball . . ."

Committee approval of a bill seldom comes easily and the rehabilitation bill was no exception. Some Committee members were not convinced there was need for the legislation, producing enough absences from Committee meetings to cause quorum problems. Others were afraid that the "physical restoration" provisions in the bill were a cover-up for a new form of socialized medicine. Resolving that one was described by Kratz years later:

"When, in our study of the text of the bill, we came to the provision for permissive physical restoration service, there was considerable opposition. Some felt it was our purpose to enter the field of social medicine, and as one put it 'They will try to cure all the sick people in Puerto Rico.' Dr. Walter Judd, a former medical missionary in China, a member of the Committee, was participating in the discussion at the time. A majority of the Committee deferred to him on this matter. That afternoon when I returned to my office, I had our files searched for a half dozen 'before and after' photographs in cases in which muscle or tendon function in a hand, arm or foot or leg had been restored or improved through physical restoration service. The next day I took these pictures to the Committee meeting and showed them to Dr. Judd. He passed them around the Committee table and said 'If that's what they want to do, I am for it.' The other members followed his lead and reversed their votes on the physical restoration provision of the bill. I am confident that if I had not convinced Dr. Judd, the bill would not have carried the provision when it came out of Committee."

Without much further delay, the Committee and the House passed the bill, and the Senate, after some generally broadening amendments, also voted its approval. On July 6, 1943 the Barden-La Follette Act was signed by President Roosevelt as Public Law 113, 78th Congress.

Now the program was equipped with a Federal law to begin making a more decisive attack on the problems of disability, both for the war period and for the future development of rehabilitation.

It was another major achievement for John Kratz. He had guided the first law into an operating program, he had been at the helm in securing the 1935 amendments, and now he had managed the enactment of a major set of changes that would influence the course of the public program for all time. Years later, when Kratz retired, Congressman Barden said: ". . . I have always felt that the rehabilitation Act should have borne his name for he was not only of valuable assistance to the Committee in preparation of the Act, but he enjoyed the absolute confidence of every man on the Committee, both Republicans and Democrats, and when in executive session, Dr. Kratz was unanimously invited into the executive sessions, and virtually every recommendation made by him was adopted."

Mr. Kratz characteristically gave much credit to others and particularly to his friend and collaborator, Mark Walter: "As President of the NRA and later as chairman of its legislative committee, he gave valuable service in the promotion of rehabilitation legislation. He was at my call to come to Washington at any time. We planned and executed strategy together, and the success of our activities in behalf of the cause of rehabilitation was due largely to his efforts and cooperation."

The course of the war was beginning to change slowly. The see-saw African campaign had given the U. S. and Allied forces control there and the movement now was to Sicily and Italy. General Patton's troops and the British-Canadian Eighth Army took Sicily July 10 and Mussolini resigned and fled. The next assault, on the Italian mainland, produced the capitulation of Italy on September 8 and, despite Nazi efforts to hold the land, the contest for this "underside" in the battle for Europe was about over. The way was slowly being cleared for the decisive assaults on France, Germany, and the Low Countries.

To the east the German Army, refusing to learn from the disaster of Napoleon, had floundered in the Russian winter and surrendered outside Stalingrad in January of 1943. From now on, on the Russian front, it would be a slow, humiliating and costly retreat westward for the Nazi troops.

In the Pacific the crucial engagements in the Coral Sea and at Midway, and the battle for Guadalcanal now were history. The Japanese fleet and its air arm had been hurt, its control of the Pacific tested and dented, but the outcome was far from decided.

On the "home front" the stringencies of a war economy were felt by everyone, often more in the little things than in the major changes—the sharply rationed gasoline and the elimination of all new automobile sales, the prices frozen under government control, "luxury" taxes on whatever non-essential goods remained, a chronic scarcity of meat, nylon stockings a special treat when they could be found. Businessmen had to get government approval to put a product into a new package, bottle or other container; restaurants stopped serving butter except on request, and not always then.

Yet in all the turmoil, people here and there could find the courage and the resources to make a beginning on something they felt strongly about. In 1943 a small clinic opened in Los Angeles to deal with the complex problems of deaf youngsters and their parents. The John Tracy Clinic, established by Mr. and Mrs. Spencer Tracy in the name of their deaf son, was incorporated with the Tracys, Walt Disney, Mrs. Orville Caldwell and Neil McCarthy as the first officers and Board members. It was perhaps the first facility to concentrate heavily on parent education as an integral part of preparing the child to master the problems of deafness. As the Clinic grew, it reached not only to families in the United States but to many in foreign countries.

In the military services, rehabilitation programs were being developed which would have a vast and prolonged influence on the whole concept of disability and its management. They emerged at an early stage of the war, particularly in the program of the Army Air Forces, and thereby averted what would have been a calamity; had the entire workload of thousands of disabled men been left to a largely unprepared Veterans Administration in the midst of the war, the result would have been chaos. The military task was formalized in a December 4, 1944 letter from President Roosevelt to Secretary of War Henry L. Stimson, directing that ". . . no overseas casualty be discharged from the armed forces until he has received the maximum benefits of hospitalization and convalescent facilities, which must include physical and psychological rehabilitation, vocational guidance, prevocational training and resocialization."

The Army Air Forces Convalescent-Rehabilitation program began as an experiment by Major Howard A. Rusk in

December of 1942 at the Jefferson Barracks Hospital in Missouri. In military service, a man was either "sick in hospital" or he was on active duty; there was no in-between period. His doctor could not send him home to take it easy for a few days.

Along with this was the wartime pressure to complete the training of all men as rapidly as possible. Major Rusk was convinced that this convalescent time should be put to practical use, both to maintain the training and skill levels of the men and to provide them with the physical reconditioning they would need to return to full duty status.

His program was brought to the attention of the Army Air Forces headquarters and, upon the recommendations of Brigadier General Hugh Morgan, the AAF placed the convalescent-rehabilitation training program in effect in all AAF hospitals. It was strongly supported by the Air Surgeon, Major General David N. W. Grant and by the Commanding General of the AAF, General H. H. ("Hap") Arnold.

The soldier-patients were made a part of their own program planning and the Air Force doctors usually functioned much like "family physicians" to aid patients with their many and varied problems.

The technical training phases of the program produced specific training aimed at the man's job in the Air Force: at Air Service Command hospitals, the program provided actual aircraft maintenance manuals, together with a variety of training aids, so that the men who were preparing to service, repair and maintain aircraft could resume their technical training and be ready to go back to their assignments when they were restored to full duty.

At Air Training Command stations, men who were preparing to be pilots, navigators, bombardiers and other flying crew members could keep up with their classes in aircraft instrumentation, navigation, oxygen systems, aerial armament and other subjects.

In all the AAF hospitals, convalescing troops were trained in such basic subjects as aircraft identification (both U. S. and allied aircraft, as well as those of the enemy), basic sanitation and health protection measures, foreign languages for areas of the world where the troops might be assigned, care and maintenance of small weapons, military map-reading and various other military subjects.

Dr. Rusk, as a colonel in the headquarters of the Air Surgeon's office in Washington, gathered about him a group of outstanding leaders to develop and direct the program. From the AAF hospitals in Miami Beach he brought Major Donald A. Covalt and Lieutenant Eugene J. Taylor to become two of his principal planners and expediters. Closely associated in developing the program was Colonel Alfred R. Shands, Jr., Chief of the Orthopedic Services of the AAF and later to be widely known as medical director of the Alfred I. du Pont Institute. Chief consultant in psychiatric care was Dr. Roy M. Grinker, directing the AAF work for the large numbers of psychiatric casualties who flowed from the intolerable pressures of war.

The AAF convalescent-rehabilitation program made extensive use of a variety of training aids, numerous special publications and motion pictures. It produced the *Handbook of Recovery* which became something of a classic in orienting ill and injured patients to the ideas and the processes of a rehabilitation program. More technical but still personalized was the crutch-walking booklet, *Let's Walk*.

Through the supply depots of the Air Service Command, a system was developed for procuring surplus supplies for the hospital program—the small handtools, items of leather and plastic, textiles and a variety of other supplies and equipment needed to carry out the program for convalescing patients. In the later stages of the war, this source of supply was made available also to the Army and Navy hospitals.

From the initial work in the small and medium-sized hospitals of the Army Air Forces, the rehabilitation program later established a series of rehabilitation centers especially equipped to provide comprehensive services for the severely disabled—the paraplegics, the psychiatric casualties, amputees and many others. One of these, at Nashville, Tennessee, was organized by Major A. Ray Dawson, who had interned at St. Elizabeth Hospital in Washington, D. C., had conducted a medical practice and who would go on to be a leading physiatrist and a specialist in designing rehabilitation programs for those recovering from mental illness.

The Army and Navy developed programs which, while differing one from the other in emphasis or detail, produced extensive rehabilitation services for their war-wounded. The Army, with its growing number of large general hospitals, established a Reconditioning Program which was able to deal successfully with the vast increase in surviving casualties which was an outstanding characteristic of World War II. For amputees there was an advanced program of care, both at Walter Reed Army Medical Center in Washington and at many other amputee centers across the country. Paraplegics and quadraplegics were cared for in large numbers for the first time in history and special centers and services were created and staffed for them. The surgical services faced all the demands of war injuries plus an increase in massive burn victims, products of bombing and armored warfare, calling not only for life-saving methods but for extended surgical procedures and prolonged rehabilitation programs.

Many of the large Army hospitals wrote chapters in military medical history, including Birmingham General at Van Nuys, Calif., Thomas England General at Atlantic

City, N. J., Woodrow Wilson General at Fishersville, Va., Percy Jones General at Battlecreek, Mich. and Valley Forge General in Pennsylvania.

The Surgeon General, Major General Norman Kirk, assigned principal responsibility for the Reconditioning program to Colonel Augustus Thorndike, who had been an early advocate of bringing medical, vocational and other efforts together in planning programs for crippled children and adults. As early as 1913, in a paper read before the orthopedic section of the New York Academy of Medicine, Dr. Thorndike had urged doctors to extend their interests beyond surgery and medication, and to direct patients into lines of training that would ready them for jobs in industry.

Like the other services, the Navy organized special rehabilitation programs for Navy and Marine victims of the war. Major hospitals and centers were focal points and these generally were located near major ports in the Navy's evacuation system. Especially heavy were the Marine casualties from the Pacific fighting as the struggle moved through the Carolines, the Marianas, and the battle for the Philippines. Under the direction of Rear Admiral Ross T. McIntire, the Surgeon General, the Navy moved from medical restorative programs into broader programs of rehabilitation and preparation for return to civilian life.

Particularly outstanding was the work done in the Mare Island Naval Hospital in California. It was to Mare Island that Dr. Henry Kessler came in October of 1943 to direct the surgical and rehabilitation work for the new amputee center. He had learned about war casualties first-hand during a year in the South Pacific combat area, most of it on the island of Efate, where casualties flowed in from Guadalcanal and other battles in often-overwhelming numbers and surgeons frequently worked around the clock. But he remembered many of his patients, despite the torrent of cases flowing in and out, and he later told many times of Case 12. This young man lost both arms, one leg and part of his jaw, plus having 60 other wounds. The surgery went on for hours and Dr. Kessler and the others had little hope the patient would survive. But as Dr. Kessler described it years later in his book, *The Knife Is Not Enough* the patient's first reaction when he came out of anaesthesia was to thank the doctors and staff for showing him so much attention. He not only lived; when Doctor Kessler saw him seven years later, he was married, had two children, a thriving insurance business and a start in politics.

At Mare Island, the Commanding Officer, Captain J. P. Owen, Dr. Douglas Toffelmeier, Captain John Greer and Dr. Kessler developed the hospital into a major amputation center, then expanded the program into psychological, educational, vocational and social programs as integral parts of the total rehabilitation service. The first stage, the artificial limb shop, did not come easily. There was no money to equip it and the usual channels for getting this done would take forever. It is customary in the military, faced with such a situation, to become a proficient "scrounger." Dr. Kessler improved on this. A local racetrack was in the financial doldrums because wartime conditions discouraged people from using their scarce gasoline ration stamps to go to the races. Dr. Kessler talked the track operators into holding a series of three "Mare Island Rehabilitation Sweepstakes", with $25,000 to go to the limb shop from each race. Business was good and, with the $75,000, the artificial limb shop got started.

To provide the professional and technical training needed to staff their programs, the armed forces turned again, as they had in a war emergency twenty-five years before, to the Institute for the Crippled and Disabled. Mr. Milbank promptly re-organized the Institute into a training in-

stitution on an emergency basis. In charge was Colonel
John N. Smith, who had become Director of the Institute
following the retirement of Dr. Faries in the mid-thirties,
and who was playing an active part in Washington in developing and pushing legislation to broaden the Federal rehabilitation law. Mrs. H. Lawrence Bogert, daughter of Mr.
Milbank, had been close to her father in the operation of
the Institute since she was a child and she put her extensive
experience to work now to help the wartime training program function smoothly. (Somehow she also found time to
work with patients at the Army's Halloran General Hospital, the Air Force Hospital at Pawling, New York, and at
Bellevue.)

The first group to seek the help of ICD was Colonel
Rusk and his Army Air Forces Convalescent-Rehabilitation
Program. Describing the training program years later, Colonel Smith pointed out: "The program established included
all of the broadened measures of physical medicine found in
the Institute's medical service. In addition, occupational therapy was expanded and there were also provided measures of
pre-vocational treatment which included shop work . . . the
accomplishment of the Air Force's program was exceptional
and highly successful. At the end of the war, it had returned
over eighty-two percent of the disabled men served to duty."

The Army and the Veterans Administration sent many
classes of trainees there. The VA groups, from sixty-nine of
its hospitals and from the Washington headquarters, usually
included an orthopedist or doctor of physical medicine, a
psychiatrist, physical therapist, occupational therapist, social worker, psychologist, vocational advisor and a training
officer.

From Canada, the Canadian Army and the Canadian
Department of Veterans Affairs sent their trainees. In 1949,
a report of the Montreal Rehabilitation Survey Committee

observed: "A striking example of the value of such a (re-habilitation) facility was the service rendered by the Insti-tute for the Crippled and Disabled during and after World War II. Because it offered extensive facilities, a well-trained staff, and a wealth of clinically-interesting material, it was able to provide rehabilitation training for United States and Canadian armed service personnel. It became a national clearinghouse for the newest in rehabilitation techniques, as well as an excellent training center for rehabilitation per-sonnel."

The ICD during the war years had an unusually gifted group of professional people. Dr. George D. Deaver, in charge of medical services, was a clinician in physical medi-cine and an exponent of functional approaches to retraining but above all, a gifted teacher. Dr. James F. Garrett, psy-chologist and counselling expert, was laying the groundwork then for later concepts in the psychological aspects of dis-ability. Miss Eleanor Brown and Miss Edith Buchwald, physical therapists, were building the idea and the proce-dures for a systematic method of teaching activities of daily living for severely injured patients. It is probable that, dur-ing the war years, students at ICD were taught more of the fundamentals of rehabilitation in a short time than any other students in history.

If there is such a thing as a "special patient", Betsy Barton was that patient at ICD during those years. A lovely girl with a personality to match, Betsy Barton at sixteen had seen her world come crashing down when she was in an auto wreck which left her a paraplegic. Her father, Bruce Barton, was widely known as an author, editor, owner of a national advertising agency and former Congressman. He also was a close friend of Jeremiah Milbank and so Betsy became a patient at ICD soon after the accident. She was a "model" patient, mastering the hard tasks of self-care and ambulation, and became an inspiration and occasional instructor for other patients. For a few years after the war, Betsy Barton was one of the more remarkable "success stories" in rehabilitation, with the publication of her books and what seemed an active and rewarding life. But Betsy died suddenly and hundreds of friends across the country mourned the loss of one of the brightest spirits in rehabilitation.

Dr. Frank Krusen was active during the war also, serving as senior consultant in physical medicine to the Army and Navy Surgeons General. At their request, he conducted intensive training courses for physicians from the two military services, who were sent to his clinic for training in physical medicine as part of the military reconditioning and rehabilitation programs. More than two hundred medical officers received training at his Department.

But the most active role he played resulted from a decision by financier Bernard M. Baruch to establish the Baruch Committee on Physical Medicine. Creation of the Committee reflected several things—Mr. Baruch's desire to memorialize his father, Dr. Simon Baruch, one of the nation's pioneers in physical medicine; his conviction that physical medicine could and should be used much more extensively to restore the war injured; and his desire to lay the groundwork for a great expansion of rehabilitation work for all disabled people.

A committee of forty scientists was named, under the chairmanship of Dr. Ray Lyman Wilbur, Chancellor of Stanford University, with Dr. Krusen as director of the Committee.

The Committee drew up a list of recommendations on priority actions that needed to be taken. It also developed model plans for rehabilitation centers and underscored the pressing need for a broader program of research in physical medicine and the equally pressing need to expand training programs for physicians and other rehabilitation personnel.

Getting on with the work, at least with the financing of it, was not difficult, according to Dr. Krusen: "We drew up a series of recommendations and then I told Mr. Baruch that we would need $1,100,000 to implement them. So he took out his checkbook and wrote a check for that amount."

In addition to numerous small grants to educational institutions around the country, the Baruch Committee made three large grants to establish major centers in teaching, research and patient care. These were made to Columbia University ($400,000), New York University ($250,000), and the Medical College of Virginia ($250,000).

From his quiet deliberations on his favorite bench in Lafayette Park opposite the White House, Mr. Baruch had helped Presidents and many others with his wise counsel, but in none of his long years of service did he help the nation more than when he built the platform from which the post–World War II rehabilitation planning was launched.

In occupational therapy and physical therapy, the war had produced a new challenge and both had responded quickly. Thanks largely to the work of Colonel Emma Vogel, the physical therapists received military status and by war's end, some 1,400 were serving in the Army. Occupational therapy had shown much the same growth; therapists were serving as key personnel in military hospitals all over the country and the total number of OT's in the country exceeded 3,000 by 1945.

Among the problems common to both the military and civilian populations was tuberculosis. In a time when drugs had not yet come to the rescue of TB patients, when millions of American military personnel abroad were subjected to old and new forms of the disease, the problems of controlling it and of rehabilitating its victims were on a very large scale. One of the first texts dealing comprehensively with rehabilitation in this field, *Occupational Therapy in the Treatment of the Tuberculosis Patient,* was published in 1944 by Miss Marjorie Fish, OTR, Director of Professional Courses in Occupational Therapy at Columbia University, and Mr. Holland Hudson, Director of the Rehabilitation Service of the National Tuberculosis Association.

By the end of 1944, the course of the war and its outcome were becoming clearer. The great Normandy invasion had carried U. S. and Allied troops to the German border and the buildup in the Pacific was slowly putting the Japanese forces into more and more defensive positions. From Port Moresby and the New Guinea staging areas, Allied troops were beginning the "island-hopping" that would bring them (and General Douglas MacArthur) back to the Philippines.

President Roosevelt, re-elected to an unprecedented fourth term in 1944, entered the spring of 1945 as the leader of the most powerful military force ever assembled. In Europe the Nazi Army was crushed and Adolf Hitler's Third Reich collapsed. Allied forces had landed at Lingayen Gulf on Luzon and begun their push into the flaming city of Manila.

But the President would not see the end, the triumph. On April 12, 1945 at his Warm Springs retreat and rehabilitation center, Franklin D. Roosevelt died. Once again, a President bearing the combined burdens of high office, a war and a severe disability, had given himself completely and without reservation to his country.

His successor in the White House faced problems the American people could not possibly comprehend. President Harry S Truman inherited more than a war that was going favorably. He faced the question of the century: to use or not to use the first nuclear weapons.

On August 5, 1945 the first atomic bomb fell on Hiroshima in Japan. Three days later the same fate was visited upon Nagasaki. On August 14 the Japanese accepted unconditional surrender.

With the end of the war, attention shifted quickly and urgently to the Veterans Administration. Just how gigantic the job was in preparing for the returning veteran had been made clear earlier in the year, when the end of the war in Europe had produced incessant demands for the discharge of personnel who had "fought their war" there. Some had been transferred to the Pacific for the final stages of the war there, but other thousands had been released from duty. Congress had provided the laws but the lack of VA personnel, new programs and money threatened a new scandal.

In the summer of 1945, General Omar Bradley, hero of the European war, was brought to Washington as the new Administrator of Veterans Affairs. With the job, he was given authority to overhaul the agency and to develop a crash program to meet the needs of the millions of veterans leaving military service. With the sudden end of the war following Hiroshima and Nagasaki, the VA job became the most pressure-laden job in Washington.

To organize the new medical service General Bradley asked for and got Major General Paul R. Hawley, who had been Bradley's chief surgeon in the European theater. Dr. Hawley, an orthopedist and a career military medical officer, had done a brilliant job of directing the medical service in Europe and had the advantage of having pulled in the same harness with General Bradley in some of the most difficult days of World War II. They made a perfect team.

The much-neglected veterans' hospitals needed to be recast into modern facilities for care of the sick and injured veteran. This called for many things—a new personnel system which would attract physicians and other health personnel into the VA medical care team, a commitment to medical research, a way to tie VA medical care into the best of American medical care elsewhere, a modernizing program for VA hospitals and a building program to produce new ones quickly, and an arrangement for bringing into the VA program the new rehabilitative ideas and methods that had evolved out of the World War II military experience.

By the end of 1945, Generals Bradley and Hawley had a new authorization from Congress, a law establishing a Department of Medicine and Surgery in the VA. On this they proceeded to build a veteran's medical care system which fulfilled the highest hopes of the President and the Congress for meeting the medical and hospital needs of the millions of returning veterans.

Dr. Hawley was surrounded with a staff of unusually talented people. In charge of research and education was Dr. Paul B. Magnuson, orthopedic surgeon of Chicago and the creator of the "Dean's Committee system" which aligned the major VA hospitals with university medical schools and their extensive teaching, research and patient care systems. In effect, the Dean's Committee arrangement gave responsibility for high quality of care for veterans to the medical schools—and the arrangement worked.

In psychiatry he had Dr. Daniel Blain and Dr. Harvey Tompkins, in tuberculosis Dr. John Barnwell, and in neurology Dr. Pearce Bailey.

A committee of consultants was named, bringing some of the most brilliant talent in American medicine into a direct and regular consulting role in the development and expansion of the veterans' hospital system.

To direct the reorganization and expansion of the medical rehabilitation service, Dr. Hawley named Dr. Donald A. Covalt, wartime associate of Dr. Howard A. Rusk. Dr. Covalt, in a matter of weeks, assembled a staff of highly expert personnel in physical medicine and rehabilitation, occupational therapy, physical therapy, prosthetics, speech pathology and audiology, specialists for the blind and in spinal cord injuries. To augment the staff, provisions were made to use personnel, most of them war-trained, in educational therapy, manual arts therapy and corrective therapy.

The VA hospital system, the largest in the world, presented a mammoth problem and a great opportunity in rehabilitation. Each of the three types of hospitals—psychiatric, tuberculosis and general—presented its own set of unique needs for specialized rehabilitation procedures. Of the three, perhaps the mental hospitals posed the most difficult problems, simply because of the deeply intrenched idea that it was all right to budget three or four dollars a day for the care of mental patients (while fifteen to twenty dollars a day was spent on patients in general hospitals). One result was a chronic and severe shortage of professional staff, making it impossible for patients to be seen very often by a psychiatrist, and reducing hospitalization largely to custodial care. It would have been worse if some of the other professionals, notably the occupational therapists, had not provided excellent diagnostic and therapeutic care. One expert, Dr. John Eisele Davis, contributed greatly in the conversion years by building into the care system his ideas on the use of sports, prescribed exercises and graduated activities programs, particularly in the treatment of schizophrenic patients.

The situation in the mental hospitals was not corrected overnight but it began to improve rapidly, mainly as a result of three factors—dynamic leadership from the top, the infusion of more Federal funds, and the influence exerted on mental hospital staffing and care by the Dean's Committee system.

In all but the smallest general hospitals, departments of physical medicine and rehabilitation were established, most of them directed by physicians with special training in the field.

A chain of spinal cord injury centers was established as one of the priority steps, with the early work done at such hospitals as the Hines (Illinois) VA hospital, the Bronx (New York) hospital, the Van Nuys (California) hospital and others.

Also at Hines was established a special center for the blind. This center represented the coordinated work between Drs. Hawley and Covalt, the VA's chief advisor on work for the blind, Warren Bledsoe, officials of the American Foundation for the Blind and numerous others. Russell Williams was named to head the Hines center for the blind and proved to be one of the most able and creative men in the history of work for the blind.

Much of the work done at Hines was the outgrowth of wartime developments in mobility training for the blind, notably the methods of Richard E. Hoover who refined the use of the cane to a near-science and used the techniques for training blind veterans at Valley Forge General Hospital in Pennsylvania.

In the VA's Vocational Rehabilitation and Education program, the pressures produced by veterans requesting services by the thousands each day reached crisis proportions by the end of 1945 and early in 1946. The main problem was recruiting and hiring competent staff fast enough to meet the onslaught of need. Numerically, the volume problem was greatest for non-injured veterans wanting education benefits under the "GI bill" but the problem of serving the disabled veteran presented its own set of problems. Military establishments, including hospitals, were being closed rapidly; there was no choice, for the doctors and other medical personnel who had staffed them were being discharged at as fast a rate as other veterans.

Harold V. Stirling, head of the Vocational Rehabilitation and Education Service, did a creditable job under the circumstances. Much of the general concepts and policies had been developed in the last two years of the war through an expert advisory committee. The cooperation of the nation's schools was sought and hundreds of colleges, universities and trade schools responded. Dr. Ira V. Scott, in charge of the counselling program of the VA, was able to establish emergency training courses for counsellors and training officers, secure the hundreds of offices needed, and convert counselling principles into practice despite the mammoth workload.

The work for disabled veterans under "PL 16" was reasonably successful but the breach between the hospitalized veteran and the VR&E program was never closed entirely. Mr. Stirling, out of his experience in the vocational rehabilitation program of World War I, when there were no veterans' hospitals and few restorative programs, found it difficult to share the rehabilitation task with the new Department of Medicine and Surgery. The result was often an administrative gap for the disabled veteran leaving the hospital and needing post-hospital rehabilitation help.

Many of the problems were minimized after Dr. James F. Garrett was recruited from the Institute for the Crippled and Disabled to head the VR&E special counselling work for disabled veterans. His in-depth experience in counselling the severely disabled and developing plans and programs for them often solved on an individual basis what was not being solved by the system.

It had become obvious, even before the end of the war, that something must be done to change the situation in artificial limbs, braces and other prosthetic devices. This "something" must include a sustained research program as well as changes in the prevailing ideas of government in purchasing and providing limbs. One of the first steps, reflecting the Army's consideration of the problem in the late stages of the war, was to set up a Prosthetics Center at Walter Reed Army Hospital in Washington.

As part of the overhauling of the Veterans Administration, it was essential that a search be started for vastly improved limbs; that limbs purchased for veterans be bought because they represented the most modern features, rather than purchasing from the lowest bidder; and that the fitting and training be under VA control and responsibility.

As a result of a Chicago conference in 1945, an advisory committee on prosthetics was established by the National Academy of Sciences-National Research Council. In November General Bradley created in the VA a Prosthetics Appliance Service, concerned with appliances and services for veterans and with the organization of a research program. Of the many scientists and technical specialists who played key roles in that period, it was Dr. Paul B. Magnuson who occupied a special position, serving both as a member of the NAS-NRC committee on prosthetics and as Director of Research and Education in the VA's Department of Medicine and Surgery.

Congress provided funds and the research program began, with contracts going to a variety of universities and industrial firms. After a year, Brig. Gen. F. S. Strong was placed in charge of the program. In 1948 the Congress passed a special law authorizing funds for prosthetics research by the VA, which selected three universities to serve as prosthetics research centers—New York University, Northwestern University and the University of California at Los Angeles. In charge of the new program was Dr. Eugene Murphy, directing the growing VA Prosthetics Center in New York City. Later the responsibility for this university-affiliated research program and for the related prosthetics education program was transferred to the Office of Vocational Rehabilitation.

In the Pentagon, where most activity was directed to "demobilization", a private preview showing of a new film was held late in 1946. The audience, mostly dignitaries and "brass" including Generals Eisenhower and Bradley, saw "The Best Years of Our Lives", the story of veterans coming back from World War II, trying to re-establish themselves in civilian life, going through that difficult process called "readjustment." (Said one of the veterans in the film, from his nook in the nose of a homeward-bound bomber: "I feel like a carburetor.")

For his starring role in "Best Years," Frederic March received an Oscar the following year. But the Academy of Motion Picture Arts and Sciences singled out one performer for two awards. Harold Russell, ex-Army sergeant and paratroop instructor who lost both hands when a defective fuse cap exploded during a training session, received an Oscar for the best supporting performance in his role as a returning injured sailor. He received the second award, a special one, for "bringing aid and comfort to disabled veterans through the medium of motion pictures."

On the fourth anniversary of Pearl Harbor, a new weekly column appeared for the first time in the Sunday *New York Times*. Dr. Howard A. Rusk, taking his wartime experience to New York City and to the nation's disabled generally, had attracted the interest of Arthur Hays Sulzburger, publisher of the *Times* who himself had some experience with, and ideas about, disability. According to Dr. Rusk, Mr. Sulzburger said at the time: "If there is anything good about war it is taking the good lessons we have learned because of war and utilizing them for the benefit of all people. I think the program developed for our disabled servicemen should be made available to all people. I would like *The*

New York Times to provide a forum for public education and national and community action toward this end." On this basis, a twenty-four-year journalistic effort on behalf of the nation's disabled began. From the beginning, reader response to the column was heavy and it quickly became evident to Dr. Rusk, to publisher Sulzburger and later to managing editor Turner Catledge that the subject of disabled people and their rehabilitation was close to the hearts of thousands of Americans in all parts of the country.

By the end of 1945, the National Foundation for Infantile Paralysis had laid its plans for a major assault on the problem of polio, including extensive plans for the rehabilitation of its victims. The Foundation, so much the child of President Roosevelt, now was in a position, with the war ended and priorities being rearranged, to launch its new program. In 1945 the Foundation committed large sums of money to several programs of research and rehabilitation. More than $1 million was provided for the general development of physical therapy programs and particularly for educational programs for therapists and fellowships for teachers in schools of physical therapy. Under the direction of Dr. Catherine Worthingham, the Foundation's Director of Professional Education, this and the other education programs soon developed into one of the most forceful programs in the post-war period for elevating and expanding rehabilitation work for polio victims and other severely disabled people.

In the following year the National Multiple Sclerosis Society was established, to form a spearhead for an organized attack on a particularly baffling neurological disease and to provide a base from which research, patient care and rehabilitation could be launched on an organized national scale.

The Federal-state program of vocational rehabilitation

had its share of post-war adjustment problems. Thousands of handicapped people who had been placed in war industries and supporting work, under relaxed job standards and simplified job operations, found themselves unemployed as industries began converting to peace-time conditions. The old bugaboo of "last on, first off" was felt widely among the handicapped. Those completing their rehabilitation programs and looking for job openings faced extremely difficult competition for a couple of years. The figures told the story: although the state rehabilitation agencies spent $5 million more in 1946 than in 1945, they rehabilitated 4,000 fewer disabled people, primarily because there were so few jobs for those ready for work. Fortunately this situation did not persist and the rehabilitation agencies, like the post-war economy generally, resumed their upward movement in 1947.

With national concern for veterans running high, many organizations and firms stepped forward with their own offers to help. One of these was the Bulova Watch Company. Arde Bulova, Chairman of the Board, had some strong personal feelings about his own and the nation's obligation to veterans. With the organizing help of his aide and Public Relations Director Colonel Harry D. Henshel, he secured the personal interest of General Omar Bradley and many others in making the Joseph Bulova School of Watchmaking a model of the manner in which private industry could help paraplegics and other disabled veterans train for skilled jobs. Their consultant and liaison to the Veterans Administration, Ben Lipton, was destined to become the widely known Director of the school in the late 1950's, and to be even more universally recognized as the "father" of wheelchair sports and a prime mover in the National Wheelchair Games and the Paralympics.

In 1947 the principal professional group in speech and

hearing changed its name to the American Speech and Hearing Association. Back in 1925 a half dozen or so early leaders in the field had formed the American Academy of Speech Correction and then, as with so many organizations, changed their name several times as the passing years and changes in concepts and practices produced new ideas. It had been that period, in fact, which moved the whole field out of the era of empiricism and personality cults, into a time of research and professional cooperation.

As the field matured, they found time to laugh. At a convention in Chicago, one of the key leaders and certainly one of the most engaging personalities in the profession, Dr. Wendell Johnson, was delivering a formal address. "Jack" Johnson, himself a victor over his own stuttering problem, had published a paper not long before in the *Quarterly Journal of Speech* pointing out that American Indians not only did not stutter, they did not even have a word for stuttering. Two of his colleagues, Dr. Jack Bangs and Dr. Harry Hollein, recruited the assistance of an authentic American Indian in full regalia, who walked up to the rostrum, in the midst of the address, and inquired loudly: "Are you the D-D-Doctor Johnson who says Indians don't st-st-st-stutter?"

Two developments in 1947 were of particular significance to the rehabilitation field. The American Board of Physical Medicine and Rehabilitation was approved, under the auspices of the American Medical Association's Advisory Board for Medical Specialties. The creation of the Board was an honor to all the pioneers who had labored for so many years to build the foundation for such a specialty—but to three of them went the signal honor of receiving the first three certificates of specialization. They were Dr. John S. Coulter, Dr. Walter J. Zeiter and Dr. Frank H. Krusen.

The other event of long range significance was the establishment in Washington of a new volunteer organization specifically aimed at promoting employment for handicapped people. Following the war a unit had been set up as the Retraining and Reemployment Administration under Marine General Graves B. Erskine, to coordinate and strengthen the Federal government's various programs for returning veterans. By 1947, it was apparent that this organization had largely completed its task for veterans and plans were made to disband it. Louis B. Schwellenbach, Secretary of Labor, proposed that for disabled veterans and disabled people generally, a special committee be established by the President to work on these problems on a long-term basis, and President Harry S Truman agreed. A Congressional resolution had been passed in 1945, largely as the work of Paul A. Strachan, President of the American Federation of the Physically Handicapped, establishing a "National Employ the Physically Handicapped Week." Two years later, with Strachan urging Schwellenbach on, the President's Committee on National Employ the Physically Handicapped Week was born. It offered a mechanism for hundreds of dedicated private citizens to work on behalf of greater employment for disabled people. First chairman of the Committee was Admiral Ross T. McIntire, former Surgeon General of the Navy before and during World War II, and former White House physician and personal physician to President Roosevelt. Named as Executive Secretary of the Committee was William P. McCahill, former newsman and Marine Corps correspondent during World War II.

The President's Committee quickly drew enthusiastic cooperation from leaders in business and industry, labor, veterans' affairs, medicine, communications,—and of course, from all spectrums of the rehabilitation "movement." It was the beginning of a long, continuous program of public education and promotion on behalf of greater employment opportunities for all handicapped people.

An active interest in rehabilitation developed in this period from an unexpected source. The United Mine Workers of America had finally achieved one of its major goals— a Welfare and Retirement Fund for miners who became disabled or who reached retirement age. The Fund had not operated very long before it was confronted with several hundred disabled miners, including many with "broken backs" from mine accidents, who needed the kind of comprehensive restorative care that seldom was available in the hospitals at that time, particularly in the coal mining regions.

The Fund quickly found that helping these miners not only was a specialized and expensive task but that few facilities in the country were capable of providing the kind of rehabilitative care required. So the Fund set up a special rehabilitation unit, conceived and directed primarily by Dr. Fred Sayers, Dr. Warren Draper and Kenneth Pohlman. Working through their regional units, the Fund found ways to locate and transport (often from isolated mountain tops) paraplegics and other disabled miners and to admit them to the few comprehensive rehabilitation centers then in existence. This program was to continue for many years and to provide service to hundreds of disabled miners who had remained outside the stream of medical care and rehabilitation.

In other places, established programs were beginning to tailor their efforts to meet the new concepts of rehabilitation for the disabled. In Chicago, the Jewish Vocational Service, which for so many years had provided a variety of vocational and related social services, acquired a new Director, Dr. William Gellman. Out of its experience with both veterans and non-veterans, the Jewish Vocational Service began a rehabilitation program which was to provide national leadership throughout the many units affiliated with the Jewish Occupational Council and which would influence workshop development generally.

In Virginia, the state rehabilitation agency was having ideas. In a demobilization period, large numbers of temporary and semi-permanent military hospitals had been closed. One of these was the Woodrow Wilson General Hospital at Fishersville, Virginia. Some of the Virginia rehabilitation staff thought it would make a perfect site for a rehabilitation center. They were convinced—from wartime experience, from the work of the Baruch Committee and from the general talk and planning within the rehabilitation fraternity— that the nation would soon see a great expansion in specialized rehabilitation centers for the disabled. To Richard Anderson, Corbett Reedy and Frank Birdsall, the vacant hospital at Fishersville represented a tremendous opportunity to provide the kind of facility they felt would be urgently needed for their handicapped clients in Virginia.

After the usual prolonged negotiations, and with the help of many people, the transfer was effected and in 1948 Mr. Birdsall was named the first supervisor of the Woodrow Wilson Rehabilitation Center.

1948 also was the year when another famous beginning was made. Dr. Howard A. Rusk opened the doors of the Institute of Rehabilitation and Physical Medicine in temporary quarters on East 38th Street in New York. The physical facility was far from ideal but the staff gathered about Dr. Rusk was enough to impress anyone. For the first nucleus there were his two wartime associates, Eugene J. Taylor and Dr. Donald A. Covalt. From the Institute for the Crippled and Disabled came Dr. George Deaver and Edith Buchwald Lawton, the latter heading the physical therapy service along with Barbara White and Tony LaRosa. Speech therapy was in the expert hands of Martha Taylor and, to head counselling psychology, Dr. James F. Garrett.

The medical staff grew with the addition of such outstanding physicians as Dr. Edward W. Lowman, Dr. Allen

Russek, Dr. Joseph Benton, Dr. Edward Gordon, Dr. Hans Kraus and Dr. Samuel Sverdlik.

In charge of rehabilitation nursing was Ellen Coffman. Her sister, Jamie Coffman, came to the Institute as a paraplegic patient and remained as one of the most valued instructors in activities of daily living. Together with Margaret Cunningham, who also came to the Institute as a patient, the two became working, living demonstrations of rehabilitation and successful living.

As the rehabilitation field grew, the National Rehabilitation Association was growing with it. In 1948 E. B. Whitten became the first full time Director of the Association, beginning a long career of leadership for the nation's fastest growing and largest organization in rehabilitation.

The following year, M. Robert Barnett was named Executive Director of the American Foundation for the Blind, succeeding Dr. Robert B. Irwin, and bringing a new vigor to the nation's best-known voluntary organization for the blind.

It was the year, too, when Dr. Henry H. Kessler realized one of his dreams. The Kessler Institute of Rehabilitation was established in West Orange, New Jersey and one of the pioneers in rehabilitation now would be able to practice the things he had been preaching so eloquently and so long. In the early stages his patients came mainly from the new rehabilitation program of the United Mine Workers, along with other patients referred from his affiliation with the Hospital for Crippled Children in Newark. A little later he recruited from the rehabilitation staff of the VA hospital at Lyons, New Jersey William K. Page as administrator of the Institute and thereby acquired one of the coming leaders in rehabilitation facility development.

Across the Hudson, Dr. Rusk and his colleagues were making plans for a new and permanent Institute. It was completed in 1950 and the world famous Institute of Rehabilitation and Physical Medicine was now ready for its long period of growth and leadership in improved patient care.

Perhaps the most important fact about the Institute in 1948 and 1949 was that it, along with so many other facilities and programs across the country, was giving tangible evidence that out of the immense tragedy of World War II, something humane and immensely beneficial was arising. The lessons, the knowledge, the convictions from World War II would not be lost.

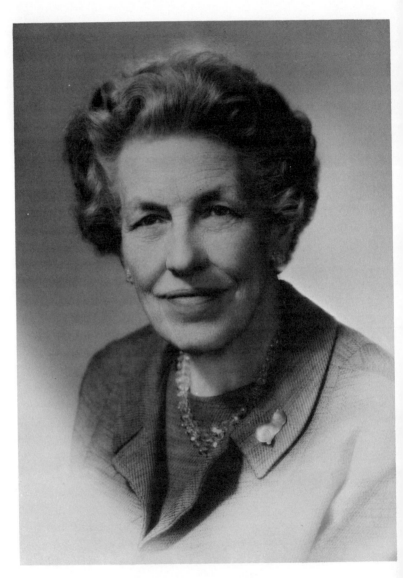

MARY E. SWITZER

CHAPTER VII

THE GROWTH YEARS

---◆◆◆◆---

THE ADVENT of a new decade always is the occasion for predictions and for second-guessing on the ten years just past. But this sort of indoor sport did not, and could not, foresee what the decade of the 1950's had in store for the development of rehabilitation programs in the United States.

It seemed, early in 1950, that another great step forward might be in the making as a result of legislation introduced by Senator Paul H. Douglas of Illinois, who had travelled the long road of rehabilitation himself after serious combat wounds as a Marine in World War II. The bill called for a new method of financing the public program, a research program, the training of personnel and several other progressive steps. Hearings were held in May of that year and the bill later passed the Senate, but the House did not act.

The loss of the Douglas bill seemed, at the time, like a major set-back. It was hard to find consolation in the fact that the Douglas bill had brought together in open forum the legislative needs of the private and public programs, that perhaps a rehearsal was necessary before the show could go on.

It was not easy to hold the attention of the public or the Congress to the Douglas bill. In June, North Korean troops invaded South Korea. The United Nations Security Council called for withdrawal of the invading troops and President Truman, announcing a "police action" in support of the UN action, sent troops into Korea. Communist troops captured Seoul and were halted only by the landing of U. S. Marines at Inchon. When more than 200,000 Chinese troops poured across the Yalu River and on into South Korea, it was easy to feel that World War III had begun.

Despite the war, there were people who pursued their ideas, plans and dreams. The "polio people" like Basil O'Connor of the National Foundation for Infantile Paralysis and the Public Health Service group and others had a dream that gamma globulin might provide the answer to a polio vaccine. Teams of workers, including the units of Lucy Blair and other physical therapists, conducted controlled studies and later carried out extensive field trials of gamma globulin.

But it would be several years and many thousands of patients before the search for a polio vaccine would be successful—and in the meantime, the rehabilitation staffs would have to keep searching for better programs for the victims of polio and the millions of others struck down with serious disabilities.

In December of 1950 Mary E. Switzer was named Director of the Office of Vocational Rehabilitation in Washington, replacing Michael J. Shortley, who became head of the Federal Security Agency's Regional Office for the middle Atlantic states.

With nearly thirty years of Federal experience, Miss Switzer took charge of a program with which she already was familiar. She had spent her earlier years with the Treasury Department where, as a member of the Secretary's staff, she had worked with the growing Public Health Service. With the transfer in 1939 of the PHS to the newly-created Federal Security Agency, Miss Switzer went to the new agency, becoming Assistant to the Administrator. In this post she had performed numerous special assignments during the war, winning the President's Award of Merit and other honors. In the post-war years she had been FSA Administrator Oscar Ewing's staff advisor for public health and for vocational rehabilitation, and thus was quite well informed on both.

The rehabilitation agency was having its problems. Relationships with the state directors of vocational rehabilitation were not particularly good. There was a financing problem with the states, arising out of the provisisons of the Federal law, which was growing more serious each year; state funds left unmatched in one year had to be provided for by setting aside funds from the next year's Federal appropriation to cover them, with this action having a snowballing effect in each successive year. Growth of the program had begun to taper off, both in the numbers rehabilitated and in the funding.

In short, at a time when rehabilitation interest and activity were blossoming in the private sector all over the country, when Federal encouragement, stimulation and help could be decisive, the Federal-state program was not in a position to help anyone.

In a matter of months, Miss Switzer began the strengthening and revitalizing of the program. Relations with state directors improved, proposals were discussed for solving the more urgent problems, and Mr. Whitten and the National Rehabilitation Association became partners in laying plans for the future. People from outside government were brought into the picture—Dr. Rusk, "Jack" Taylor, Drs. Krusen and Kessler, Lawrence Link and Jayne Shover of the National

Society for Crippled Children, Col. John Smith of the Institute for the Crippled and Disabled in New York, Dr. Warren Draper of the United Mine Workers' Welfare and Retirement Fund, Bell Greve in Cleveland and Peter Salmon of the Industrial Home for the Blind in Brooklyn—all of them and others becoming official or unofficial advisors.

In mid-spring of 1951 a meeting was held with Arthur S. Flemming, Assistant to the Director in the Office of Defense Mobilization, the government's principal planning and control arm for the Korean emergency. Dr. Rusk, as Chairman of the Health Resources Advisory Committee, reported both to President Truman and Mr. Flemming in carrying out the "doctor draft" law and in various related health policy issues. Dr. Rusk, Miss Switzer and Dr. Theodore G. Klumpp, President of Winthrop-Stearns, Inc., a drug firm, and former government official, discussed with Mr. Flemming the emergency manpower problems in the Korean war and how the rehabilitation program might help with them.

The result was the establishment in May, 1951, of an ODM Task Force on the Handicapped to review the Federal-state and other rehabilitation programs in light of war emergency needs and propose steps which the government and others should take to develop rehabilitation programs so that maximum use could be made of handicapped manpower.

Named to the Task Force were Dr. Daniel Blain, Medical Director of the American Psychiatric Association; Colonel E. W. Palmer, President of the Kingsport Press in Tennessee, a Director of the National Association of Manufacturers and a volunteer leader of the National Society for Crippled Children and Adults; Dr. George D. Deaver, Professor of Clinical Physical Medicine and Rehabilitation at New York University-Bellevue Medical Center; Dr. Carroll L. Shartle, Professor of Psychology at Ohio State University and officer of the American Psychological Association; Davis B. Geiger, official of the Ben Williamson Company and President of the National Society for Crippled Children and Adults; Dr. M. D. Mobley, Executive Secretary of the American Vocational Association; Dr. Dorothy C. Stratton, National Executive Director of the Girl Scouts of the U. S. A. and a wartime National Director of the SPARS; Frank L. Fernbach, Associate Director of Research for the CIO and Vice President of the American Federation of the Physically Handicapped; Dr. Charles S. Wise, Professor of Physical Medicine and Rehabilitation at George Washington University Medical School; and Henry Viscardi, Jr., Executive Director, JOB (Just One Break) and faculty member of the New York University College of Medicine.

Consultants to the Task Force were Mary Switzer; Arthur S. Motley, Assistant Director of the Bureau of Employment Security in the Department of Labor; and Dr. Vern K. Harvey, Medical Director of the U. S. Civil Service Commission.

The Task Force was further supported by a joint secretariat composed of experts from several government agencies—the Department of Labor, the Federal Security Agency, the Public Health Service and the U. S. Civil Service Commission. Especially active in assisting the Task Force were Earl T. Klein, Consultant on Selective Placement with the U. S. Employment Service, and K. Vernon Banta, Assistant Executive Secretary of the President's Committee on National Employ the Physically Handicapped Week.

In early 1952 the Task Force submitted its report and a set of twenty-two recommendations, including proposals for action at the local, state and national levels. The group proposed steps to survey and expand training and employment resources for the handicapped, to increase funds for the Federal-state program, to train more professional workers including team training, and to conduct a national inventory of rehabilitation facilities.

The Task Force report had many direct effects, such as the four-year study-and-service-program carried out in the metropolitan Kansas City area, sponsored by the Kansas City Association of Trusts and Foundations, under the direction of Homer Wadsworth, Dr. Carroll Bryant and Dr. Eleanor Poland, with the cooperation of Joy Talley, Missouri State Director of Vocational Rehabilitation. But the report had a longer-range effect, by becoming a factor in the development of legislative plans which culminated in the 1954 amendments to the Federal rehabilitation law.

One of the recommendations—regarding facilities—received prompt attention, mainly as a result of the prodding and persevering of Henry Redkey, facilities specialist in OVR. (In fact, it was his missionary work which helped convince the Task Force that something must be done in the facility field.)

On October 29, 1951 Redkey wrote a memorandum to Mary Switzer, pointing to the rising activities in centers and workshops, and to the nearly-complete absence of national information on facilities. He urged the convening of a conference of facility people, to lay the groundwork for gathering information and to begin developing some criteria and standards for the development and improvement of centers.

It was the following August before a Steering Committee was named, bringing together Redkey, Dr. Joseph H. Gerber, Bell Greve, Jayne Shover and Eugene J. Taylor to draft the preliminary plans for the conference. A program was put together with great care, with the help of people like William Stearns, William Page, June Sokolov of the Hartford County Rehabilitation Workshop in Connecticut, Vivian Shepherd of the Rehabilitation Institute in Kansas City and Willis Gorthy, Associate Director of the Institute for the Crippled and Disabled.

On December 1, 1952 the conference was convened in Indianapolis, with Roy Patton, Director of the Crossroads Rehabilitation Center there, serving as host. The great variation in the types of rehabilitation facilities was apparent: from the Ohio State University Rehabilitation Center came Dr. Ralph Worden, Director, and Kenneth Hamilton, Assistant Director; from Goodwill Industries came Dayton executive Lee H. Lacy and Cincinnati executive Bryce W. Nichols; from the state-operated center at Fishersville, Virginia there was Frank Birdsall; Marjorie Taylor of the Curative Workshop of Milwaukee and Colonel Smith and Willis Gorthy of ICD contributed from their long experience; and from the Delaware Curative Workshop there was Eleanor J. Bader.

For the OVR in Washington there was, in addition to Redkey, Mary Switzer, Dr. James Garrett, Tracy Copp and two of the senior regional representatives, John H. Lasher and Tom G. Rathbone. For the National Rehabilitation Association there was E. B. Whitten.

Out of the Indianapolis meeting came a shaky new organization, the Conference of Rehabilitation Centers, with Willis Gorthy of ICD as first President. Progenitor of the Association of Rehabilitation Centers, it would in turn become, through a merger with the National Association of Sheltered Workshops and Homebound Programs, the facility organization of the '70's, the International Association of Rehabilitation Facilities.

The stirring around in Washington on so many health and rehabilitation fronts in 1951 produced another effort to effect some changes. In December, President Truman appointed a Commission on the Health Needs of the Nation, with Dr. Paul B. Magnuson as Chairman. Among the distinguished group of members were Dr. Russel V. Lee, Director of the Palo Alto Clinic in California; Albert J. Hayes, President of the International Association of Machinists; Walter P. Reuther, President of the United Auto Workers; Marion W. Sheahan, R. N., of the National League for Nursing; Dr. Lowell J. Reed, of Johns Hopkins University; Dr. Evarts A. Graham, Professor of Surgery at Washington University; Chester I. Barnard, Chairman of the National Science Foundation; and Charles S. Johnson, President of Fisk University.

In addressing itself to national health policies and proposing a course for health care, the Magnuson Commission called attention to needs and opportunities in rehabilitation throughout its report. Much of this was the result of the Commission's Panel on Rehabilitation, for which Miss Switzer served as a keynoter, and whose membership included Dr. Alexander P. Aitken, Professor of Clinical Orthopedic Surgery at Tufts College of Medicine, Dr. Ben Boynton of the Veterans Administration PMR staff, Dr. Warren Draper of the United Mine Workers, F. Ray Power, West Virginia State Director of Vocational Rehabilitation, Dr. Rusk, Peter Salmon, and others.

Four major recommendations regarding rehabilitation were made by the Magnuson Commission—a substantial increase in the numbers of personnel trained in rehabilitation, the orientation of all health personnel to the concept of "total care", the development of far more rehabilitation departments in general hospitals and the establishment of additional specialized rehabilitation centers, and the expansion of the Federal-state vocational rehabilitation program.

The impact of the Commission on national health care thinking and planning at that time was reduced by an event having nothing to do with health care: its report to President Truman, submitted December 18, 1952, came more than two months after Dwight D. Eisenhower had been elected President of the United States. Thus the report to a Democratic President was inherited by a new Republican President and a Republican Congress.

Although the Commission recommendations did not become official grist for the new Administration's mill, President Eisenhower and his advisors moved very quickly in the fields of health and education and welfare. One of the first major accomplishments of the new Administration was the creation of a Department of Health, Education and Welfare in April, 1953, aided notably by Senator Robert A. Taft of Ohio in guiding it through the Congress.

For practical purposes, the new Department was a reframing of the old Federal Security Agency, yet in the unwritten laws of the bureaucracy, health and education and welfare became major elements in the nation's business when they became a Department.

Named as first Secretary of the new Department was Mrs. Oveta Culp Hobby of Houston, with Nelson Rockefeller as Under Secretary.

Soon after creation of the Department, there were discussions and plans for the development of legislation to amend the Vocational Rehabilitation Act. Secretary Hobby and Under Secretary Rockefeller were dealing with a President who had had considerable experience with disability and rehabilitation. He had learned from his broad military experience about the problems of disability and about the programs developed for disabled veterans. As President of Columbia University following the war, he had served on the board of the Institute for the Crippled and Disabled and had had many other personal contacts with organizations concerned with disabled people.

In the new Republican Congress, the House Committee on Education and Labor acquired a new Chairman, Samuel K. McConnell, Jr. of Pennsylvania. Sitting also as Chairman of a Special Subcommittee on Assistance and Rehabilitation of the Physically Handicapped, Mr. McConnell conducted hearings in 1953 into the vocational rehabilitation program and related matters affecting the handicapped. Although the Administration had not yet proposed legislation, Miss Switzer appeared before the Subcommittee and testified to the general lines of legislation that would be most helpful.

The Committee was subjected to a ridiculous amount of bickering, both internally and externally. Congressman Graham Barden, former Chairman of the full Education and Labor Committee and co-author of the 1943 Barden–La Follette Vocational Rehabilitation Act, did not take kindly to his role as ranking minority member. Although he had given little time and attention to improving the Vocational Rehabilitation Act or its program since the 1943 Act, he exhibited strong paternal feelings about the program and obviously was not happy that a Republican Congress was about to make changes in a law which bore his name. During later sessions, he twice stalked in anger from the Committee room. Another Democrat, Congressman Roy Wier, regularly led the discussions into a corner with pointless questions.

Paul A. Strachan wanted to set up a new agency to encompass all Federal programs and activities related to handicapped people. Dr. Jacobus Ten Broek of the National Federation of the Blind castigated the OVR for a variety of deficiencies and tangled with representatives of the American Foundation for the Blind, principally over proposals to amend the Randolph-Sheppard Act.

But Sam McConnell was a man of unlimited patience and an equal amount of determination to get a good bill.

He had constructive help from both sides of the political aisle, notably from Democratic Congressman Carl Perkins of Kentucky and Republican Congressman John Rhodes of Arizona. Too, most leaders in rehabilitation, in and out of government, had been deep into the questions of legislative needs for some time, as a result of the Douglas bill hearings, the work of the Task Force, NRA meetings and other activities, so that the general nature of the 1954 amendments was becoming fairly clear.

The interest in Federal legislation was interrupted in November of 1953 with the death of Col. John N. Smith, Director of the Institute for the Crippled and Disabled. His work there, his important role in the young facilities movement and his personal commitment to rehabilitation had made him widely known and respected among rehabilitation workers. At a ceremony conferring a special posthumous award on him by the President's Committee on Employment of the Physically Handicapped, Jeremiah Milbank said: "I admired Colonel Smith and had a deep affection for him as a friend. It was my privilege twenty years ago to select him as Director of the Institute. I never knew a man who so quickly grasped every opportunity to help the handicapped . . ."

The legislation which the Administration sent to the Congress late in 1953 was constructive in its content and it received priority in the work schedule of Congress. The new Department of HEW gave the legislation its full attention when House hearings were resumed. The Under Secretary Nelson Rockefeller and his assistant, Rod Perkins, put in many hours on many days developing data, converting it to charts and making effective presentations before the House committee. Backed up by Director Mary Switzer, and by long days of dedicated labor by Assistant Director Donald H. Dabelstein, the HEW team functioned with great efficiency. The House Committee, with the benefit of its prior hearings, went into executive session and, with the help of agency officials and many representatives of private organizations, thrashed out a bill which passed the House with virtually no objections.

In the Senate, the process was briefer and easier. Senator William Purtell of Connecticut, Chairman of the Health Subcommittee of the Senate Committee on Labor and Public Welfare, held hearings and reported a bill which was much closer to what the Administration had asked for than was the House-passed bill. It passed the Senate in the late spring of 1954 without difficulty.

The Senate-House conferees had little difficulty reconciling the two bills and on August 3, 1954 President Eisenhower signed Public Law 565, 83rd Congress, the "Vocational Rehabilitation Act Amendments of 1954."

It was more than another Federal law on the books in Washington. The 1954 Act recast the role of the Federal government in advancing rehabilitation work for the disabled in the United States. It established the basis for a realistic working partnership between public and private organizations in improving and expanding rehabilitation. It made provision for more funds and additional program devices for the state vocational rehabilitation agencies. It inaugurated a new Federally-assisted research program for both private and public agencies; it accepted a Federal responsibility to help increase the numbers of professional and technical people trained to staff the private and public programs; it authorized grants to expand, alter and improve facilities.

Thus the Congress put together in one cohesive set of programs in one place the essential elements for progressive and successful rehabilitation work for disabled people, the elements that rehabilitation leaders had been seeking for more than thirty years.

The plans for the new research program were modelled generally along the operating lines of the National Institutes of Health, and provided for a National Advisory Council on Vocational Rehabilitation to help establish policy and to provide expert, non-governmental review of research grant applications. The "founding" members of the Council were an interesting blend of backgrounds, brought together with experienced rehabilitation professionals to provide a balanced mix of "the public interest" and the "pros." Included were Voyle Scurlock, State Director of the vocational rehabilitation program in Oklahoma and one of the senior leadership figures in the public program; Dr. Henry Kessler; Eli Gorodezky, prominent attorney and civic leader in Phoenix; Dr. Frank H. Krusen; Peter J. Salmon; Mrs. Spencer Tracy of the John Tracy Clinic in Los Angeles; Dr. Theodore G. Klumpp of New York, drug company official and Chairman of the 1951 Task Force on the Handicapped; Chester W. Haddan, nationally-known prosthetic expert of Denver; Russell W. Brothers, Nashville businessman; and Henry Viscardi, Jr., now President of Abilities, Inc. on Long Island.

The rehabilitation-minded Congress in 1954 did more. They passed an amendment to the Social Security Act to protect those workers who became disabled, by "freezing" their benefits at the level they had earned when they became disabled; thus, without further payments into the system, they would, when they became 65, have their retirement income benefits. To examine those who applied for the disability "freeze" benefits, the Congress indicated the state rehabilitation agencies as the agency-of-choice, and nearly all states selected the rehabilitation agency for the job. The law also called for the state agencies to consider each applicant for his rehabilitation potential and to restore him to employment if possible. Thus began an official working relationship between vocational rehabilitation and the Social

Security program, one which would assume larger proportions when the Social Security program later expanded into disability cash benefits and still later into using Social Security funds to pay for vocational rehabilitation services to the System's beneficiaries.

It was the year, also, when the Hill-Burton hospital construction law was amended to authorize a new, separate grant program to help build more rehabilitation facilities, principally those in hospitals and other medical and health settings.

Getting the vocational rehabilitation bill enacted in mid-summer was fortunate, for 1954 was a Congressional election year and by fall, much of Washington's attention had turned to the coming November contests throughout the country. President Eisenhower's popularity was high and the chances of retaining Republican control in both the House and Senate appeared good. But the normally Democratic districts, plus the so-called "right to work" issue fought strenuously by organized labor in many districts, gave control of the Congress back to the Democrats, to remain that way for a long time.

In Minneapolis the Mayo Memorial Hospital officially activated its new University of Minnesota Rehabilitation Center in 1954, beginning the story of one of the nation's foremost research, teaching and patient care facilities. Getting the center into being reflected the support of many local professional and civic groups; even the Mayor, Hubert H. Humphrey, as Chairman of the Mayor's Committee on Employment of the Handicapped, had put his shoulder to that particular wheel.

Next door in Wisconsin, Marjorie Taylor ended her long and successful service as Executive Director of the Curative Workshop of Milwaukee and was succeeded by Tore Allegrezza.

In New York, the two-year-old business venture called Abilities, Inc. was facing the future with fingers crossed. Henry Viscardi, Jr. and Art Nierenberg had decided in 1952 that they could and would start a commercial business staffed entirely with severely handicapped people—and make it pay. So far, they had succeeded; the working force had grown from four to sixty and the volume of business was holding strong. But the end of the Korean war was just around the corner and the defense orders which were a sizeable part of Abilities' business would begin tapering off when the conflict ended.

It was a period which helped transform Abilities from a highly idealistic gamble into a progressive, hard-headed enterprise which learned to anticipate and weather many changing business conditions and still prove its original point—that severely disabled people can compete and produce successfully in the free enterprise system. Viscardi and his associates did more than survive the transition; they made plans for a large new building to house a bigger dream, a Human Resources Center where the industrial work could be expanded and aligned with a school for severely disabled children and a work-oriented research laboratory.

Another New Yorker was spotlighted in 1955 when Dr. Arthur S. Abramson was named Handicapped American of the Year by the President's Committee on Employment of the Physically Handicapped. If the Committee's protocol for awards had permitted it, the Committee probably would have named him Physician of the Year as well, for Abramson was a part of the "new breed" that was bringing new scientific and clinical stature to the specialty of physical medicine and rehabilitation. Victim of a World War II combat injury, Abramson had demonstrated that a paraplegic could not only master a career in medicine but could become one of its leaders.

There was a rising tide of rehabilitation interest in international activities to encourage and help expand rehabilitation programs abroad. Much of this effort was directed into the activities of the International Society for the Welfare of Cripples which offered an experienced mechanism by which professionals in the United States could collaborate with their peers abroad.

There was no means of providing any substantial financial aid for such international rehabilitation work except for the limited rehabilitation interests of the World Health Organization and the more established interests and activities of the International Labor Organization.

In 1955 Dr. Rusk and his associate Eugene J. Taylor were instrumental in establishing the World Rehabilitation Fund as a voluntary organization primarily interested in supporting the training of physicians and other professionals in rehabilitation techniques, as a means of establishing nuclei of rehabilitation work in many countries abroad. The Fund also was much interested in advancing research and gave its aid to the establishment of programs and facilities in numerous places. Dr. Rusk had begun to be active in such international work earlier when the American Korean Foundation was established and he made his first mission to Korea for the President in 1953. Founding Chairmen of the World Rehabilitation Fund were Bernard M. Baruch, former Presidents Herbert Hoover and Harry S Truman, and Dr. Albert Schweitzer.

In Los Angeles, the county hospital, Rancho Los Amigos, took advantage of its extensive experience with polio patients and broadened its work to establish an intensive treatment program for the severely disabled generally. Rancho Los Amigos, begun in 1887 as a county poor farm, had later evolved into a hospital for the care of long-term chronic disease patients and then, in 1944, had become one of the early respirator centers for polio patients. In 1952 the National Foundation for Infantile Paralysis and the County of Los Angeles provided the first funds to establish a combination respiratory and rehabilitation center for polio patients and Rancho Los Amigos found itself deep into the problems of the severely disabled victims of polio. The decision in 1955 to move into the problems of other severe disabilities led the way to making Rancho Los Amigos one of the outstanding rehabilitation centers in the United States.

The transformation attracted an orthopedic surgeon who would make Rancho a major part of his professional career. Dr. Vernon L. Nickel had had some brief exposures to rehabilitation ideas and programs during World War II and afterward but it had not "taken." Many years later, in delivering the Sir Robert Jones Lecture at the Hospital for Joint Diseases and Medical Center in New York City, he noted that ". . . This experience did not in any way induce me to become interested or involved in orthopedic rehabilitation until, by pure happenstance, I began working at Rancho Los Amigos Hospital with my classmate, Dr. John Affeldt, an outstanding internist and respiratory physiologist . . . At Rancho I became stimulated and excited by the tremendous professional challenges and opportunities equalling or surpassing the satisfactions of caring for patients with more conventional problems."

This was the story of many professional people who "found their way" into rehabilitation. They came, and continue to come, for a mix of highly personalized reasons—keen professional interest, strong personal convictions about the problems of disability, reaction to challenge—and perhaps some of the same dedication which brings people into the serving professions in the first place.

In 1956 the Cleveland Rehabilitation Center merged with the Vocational Guidance Bureau to form a new center and service organization, the Vocational Guidance and Re-habilitation Services. Chosen as the executive for the new organization was Mrs. Olive Kennedy Bannister, who had been instrumental in creating the Vocational Guidance Bu-reau and who would become one of the best known and most able center executives in the country.

This was the same year that the President's Commit-tee on Employment of the Handicapped learned the hard way about architectural barriers for the handicapped. Hugo Deffner, Oklahoma City insurance man and himself severely handicapped, had been one of the first people in the country to conduct a sustained campaign against architectural bar-riers and he had been hard at work on his self-elected mis-sion for ten years. In 1956 the President's Committee se-lected Deffner as the "Handicapped Man of the Year" for his architectural barriers battle.

It proved an embarrassing time for the President's Committee. The Departmental Auditorium of the Depart-ment of Labor, where the meeting and the ceremonies were held, had steps—lots of steps—and Hugo Deffner and his wheelchair had to be carried into the building to be honored for his fight against architectural barriers. (He was scarcely out of town before workmen were on the job, making the Departmental Auditorium "barrier free.")

One of the most interesting personalities to "invade" the rehabilitation field came along in 1956 in the person of Dr. Allen H. Eaton. Dr. Eaton, an author, scholar and cul-tural expert, talked with OVR Director Mary Switzer about his ideas of encouraging communication between sighted and blind people through the enjoyment of beauty. More specifically, he believed that various art objects and small sculptures could, through their form, texture and lines create an artistic satisfaction for the blind and equally for the sighted. Working with the OVR, the American Foundation for the Blind and others, he developed a portable collection of forty-one art objects. It included such varied items as a prehistoric stone hand tool from France, a carved ebony giraffe, a Babylonian clay tablet bearing cuneiform inscription, a two and one half inch crystal sphere, cut from natural quartz, and Toscanini's favorite baton, a slender birch pointer with a cork handle and ferrules of moss green and coral plastic.

Dr. Eaton's ideas and his inspiring art objects were put between the covers of an illustrated book *Beauty for the Sighted and the Blind* in 1959. Later, in the 1960's the North Carolina Museum of Art used Dr. Eaton's concepts to develop a permanent exhibit, establishing the Mary Duke Biddle Gallery for the Blind, opened in 1966. Similar exhibits were established at the Hartford, Connecticut Wadsworth Atheneum and at the Brooklyn Museum. The California State Art Commission developed both a traveling exhibit and a gallery.

At the Institute for the Crippled and Disabled in New York, now in a new period of growth under the direction of Willis Gorthy, a new method of evaluating the aptitudes and work capacities of the seriously disabled was introduced.

Called the TOWER system (Testing, Orientation, and Work Evaluation in Rehabilitation) it was the product of many ICD staff members, primarily Jay O'Brien and Donald G. Weiss, the latter the Institute's Director of Public Relations and New York public relations expert. The TOWER system and its extensive materials, produced for center and workshop use, provided one of the first formalized methods of visualizing and using a variety of work sample techniques in the early stages of testing and planning for the handicapped client.

In the last half of the Fifties, honors began to flow to some of the leaders who had influenced rehabilitation so remarkably. Dr. Frank Krusen received the 1956 *Modern Medicine* Award for Distinguished Achievement; the American Heart Association conferred the Howard W. Blakeslee Award for medical science writing on Eugene J. Taylor for his series in *The New York Times* on cardiovascular defects (a series published not long after President Eisenhower's heart attack); and the American Congress of Physical Medicine and Rehabilitation bestowed its prestigious Gold Key Award on Dr. Miland Knapp (now looking back with some nostalgia on the rigors of his early practice in the Thirties). At the Seventh World Congress of the International Society for the Welfare of Cripples in London in 1957, Dr. Howard Rusk was honored with the Albert Lasker Award for his massive contributions to rehabilitation both at home and internationally. The following year he received the Physician's Award of the President's Committee. In 1959 the Committee selected a widely-known California physician in rehabilitation, Dr. John H. Aldes, Director of the Rehabilitation Center at the Cedars of Lebanon Hospital in Los Angeles.

Two of the quietly strong, devotedly aggressive people were lost to rehabilitation in the late 1950's. Bell Greve, early proponent of rehabilitation programs, Director of the Cleveland Rehabilitation Center, long-time Secretary of the International Society for the Welfare of Cripples, and Director of Welfare for the City of Cleveland under Mayor Anthony Celebrezze, died in 1957. The following year the Office of Vocational Rehabilitation in Washington lost its creative program planner and something of its character when Donald H. Dabelstein, Assistant Director of OVR and one-time rehabilitation counselor in the state program in Minnesota, died.

The Institute for the Crippled and Disabled in New York had an unusual trainee in 1958. The life story of President Franklin D. Roosevelt, told in the book *Sunrise at Campobello,* was about to become a stage play and a movie. Ralph Bellamy, preparing to star in the role of F.D.R. came to ICD for three weeks of exhausting training to learn to live the life of a paraplegic on crutches and braces, to maneuver a wheel chair, and to think like a victim of polio.

In Pennsylvania, where the vocational rehabilitation program had developed into one of the nation's largest and best, the new state director, Charles L. Eby, had the pleasure of opening a new center at Johnstown in 1959. The facility marked the first time that a large, comprehensive vocational rehabilitation center had been designed and built by a state agency. Named as first Director of the Center was Charles L. Roberts, whose career would take him later to the post of Executive Vice President of the International Association of Rehabilitation Facilities.

By the late stages of the 1950's it was apparent that the experimental days, the proving period of rehabilitation was over. In all directions, in all parts of the nation, new programs were springing up, old programs were growing larger. Federal and state funds had increased sharply, the voluntary fund raising organizations were expanding, the numbers of disabled rehabilitated had risen steadily, the Federally-aided research and training programs were solidly established and productive, and facilities were increasing.

The diversity was as interesting as the volume. In New York a successful businessman, Thomas D'Arcy Brophy, Chairman of the Board of the Kenyon and Eckhardt advertising agency and himself the victim of severe burns, joined with Dr. Rusk and Dr. John Marquis Converse, Director of the Institute of Reconstructive Plastic Surgery at New York University Medical School, to help establish a Society for the Rehabilitation of the Facially Disfigured.

In California, Justin Johnson, official of the Hughes

Aircraft Company and Chairman of the California Governor's Committee on Employment of the Handicapped, was becoming a one-man national movement in spurring jobs for handicapped men and women throughout the country.

In Washington, the long-standing jurisdictional bickering between the Department of Labor and the Department of HEW was being quieted by the performance and personality of James P. Mitchell, Secretary of Labor. Impatient with quarrels over control of various Federal agencies (most of which went back to the government organizations of the New Deal days in the 1930's), Jim Mitchell's attitude and technique were demonstrated one evening when he arrived late for a speech before HEW's Regional Directors in the Willard Hotel and opened his remarks with: "I don't know what you gentlemen have been talking about this evening, but if you're talking about trading agencies, I have a couple I'd like to *give* you."

In Minnesota several of the medical leaders in rehabilitation created a new nonprofit organization, the American Rehabilitation Foundation. The Foundation was the outgrowth of a scandal that had descended on the Kenney Institute as a result of the manipulation of funds by an employee, threatening the integrity and even the existence of the Institute. Dr. Krusen, asked to lead the efforts to rescue the center and restore public confidence, gave two years to the task. The Institute's affairs were untangled and the Foundation was established with wide community, state and national support. The Foundation, however, served a broader purpose than this. As a mechanism for the future, it reflected the rehabilitation experience and the aims of Dr. Krusen, Dr. Frederic Kottke, Dr. Paul Ellwood and others associated with the University of Minnesota and the Kenney Rehabilitation Institute. Through the Foundation and its several Expert Committees, it was possible to merge into a sustained research effort the medical, psychological, vocational and other aspects of rehabilitation progress. As their respective roles developed, the University of Minnesota faculty emphasized clinical research, with the Foundation efforts going in the direction of research on the delivery of health services, quality controls and clinical applications.

At the famed center at Warm Springs, Georgia, a new dimension was added with the construction of a large vocational rehabilitation center by the Georgia state rehabilitation agency. The two units, functioning together as a comprehensive center for the disabled, more or less formalized the close working relations which had been developed many years before between one of Georgia's early State Directors, Paul Barrett and by his successor, A. Polk Jarrell. Their work with the medical staff at Emory University at Atlanta, and particularly with Dr. Robert Bennett, a leading physiatrist of Emory and Medical Director at Warm Springs, had been a prime factor in the large amount of restorative work done for the disabled by the Georgia agency and in placing the Georgia program at the top of the list for many years in the numbers of disabled rehabilitated annually.

In 1960 the Vocational Rehabilitation Administration in the Department of HEW established its first international rehabilitation program. The program developed from VRA's negotiations within the government for authority to use excess U. S.-owned foreign currencies in other countries to finance rehabilitation research and demonstration programs abroad. As this plan was nearing completion, the Congress passed the "Health for Peace" Act, providing for use of both foreign currencies and U. S. dollars to conduct foreign health and rehabilitation research. Combined with the domestic authority, the VRA now was ready to work with many countries abroad.

In record time, regulations and guidelines were published, making it possible for Miss Switzer and the VRA staff to discuss plans and projects with foreign representatives during the Eighth World Congress of the International Society for the Welfare of Cripples, held for the first time in the United States in New York City in August 1960. It was at that World Congress that the ISWC became the Internationl Society for Rehabilitation of the Disabled, formalizing the commitment of dozens of countries to rehabilitation as a modern approach to the problems of disability.

A close working partner with the new international rehabilitation program was the World Rehabilitation Fund, now well-established and experienced in the field. Impressed with the tremendous need for better artificial limbs and braces in so many parts of the world, and particularly in the underdeveloped countries, Dr. Rusk and Mr. Taylor of the Fund undertook a sustained campaign to do something about the situation. Their emissary, Juan Monros, a native of Spain and U. S.-trained, became perhaps the only expert in rehabilitation to devote his entire career to travel abroad, conducting training courses in prosthetics and orthotics in dozens of countries and helping many nations to organize and operate their own shops and services.

In November 1960 the American voters elected John F. Kennedy as the thirty-fifth President of the United States. While his electoral vote margin over Republican Richard M. Nixon was substantial, he carried the popular vote by a thin line of slightly over 100,000.

President Kennedy brought into the office with him a sense of youthful vigor, of refreshed confidence in the future. Not even a snow storm which paralyzed the city of Washington on the evening of his inauguration dimmed the enthusiasm. The 1960's began as a decade brimming with optimism.

In his first year in the White House, President Kennedy

threw the full weight of his office and prestige behind a dramatic effort to confront and master the problems of mental retardation. The Kennedy family had lived with the problem, through the eldest daughter who was retarded. They knew that only a frontal attack on the public consciousness could begin to erase some of the deeply implanted myths about retarded people; only a powerful and sustained push could arouse professionals to the research, the program-building, and the coordinated efforts that would produce new scientific information, prevent unnecessary retardation, distinguish between pathologic retardation and the results of deprivation, and provide happier and more useful lives for its victims.

The attack on mental retardation was a family affair— the parents, former Ambassador and Mrs. Joseph P. Kennedy; brothers Robert F. Kennedy, the new Attorney General, and Edward M. Kennedy; Sargent Shriver and Mrs. Eunice Kennedy Shriver. As a rallying point, a President's Committee on Mental Retardation was formed. The job would have been far more difficult if there had not been a young, vital and fast-growing National Association for Retarded Children. The NARC was a product of the coming together of parents seeking strength in their search for help for their retarded youngsters. It provided the sort of grass-roots organization that could bring to life the quiet desperation of thousands of Americans struggling with the problems of retardation.

The government agencies responded quickly. Mary Switzer and the Vocational Rehabilitation Administration in HEW began developing special projects and program goals, with the state rehabilitation agencies giving their prompt support. The VRA had tried before in mental retardation. Back in the Fifties, psychologist Dr. Salvatore DiMichael had urged, in the professional literature and in programming, that far more be done to provide rehabilitation services and jobs for the retarded. Miss Switzer had promoted the idea that rehabilitation programs should devote more of their time, talents and money to restoring the retarded and the mentally ill. Many state agencies had accepted the challenge and some experience already was accumulated. Now the time had come for moving against retardation on a broad front.

Other government agencies joined. The President's Committee on Employment of the Physically Handicapped pin-pointed mental retardation and mental illness as special targets for the committee's efforts to clear away misunderstandings and open up employment opportunities. (President Kennedy later shortened the Committee's name by dropping the word "Physically".) The Chairman, retired Marine Major General Melvin J. Maas, himself blind and a veteran of World Wars I and II (and of the Congressional wars as a former Congressman from Minnesota) gave strong leadership to the new program. First the Executive Secretary, William McCahill, became the operating wedge; later his Deputy, Bernard Posner, made the cause of the retarded and the mentally restored a crusade. The U. S. Civil Service Commission took the first steps to change its hiring procedures to bring more retarded people into a wider range of jobs they could do. The U. S. Employment Service in the Department of Labor worked out new plans with the state employment agencies to fit the retarded into more community employment.

Legislation was sent to Congress to create new programs in mental retardation and strengthen several existing ones. The first tangible result came with enactment of the Mental Retardation Facilities and Community Mental Health Centers Construction Act of 1963 which, with its subsequent amendments, provided the Federal springboard for a major national effort. Many states passed their own legislation, both to join in the Federal programs and to carry out their own plans.

President Kennedy's interest was not confined to the rehabilitation needs of the mentally retarded. On a beautiful August day in 1962 he greeted HEW Secretary Anthony Celebrezze, Commissioner Switzer and others in the Rose Garden of the White House for a special occasion. Figures just in from the states showed that the state vocational rehabilitation agencies had rehabilitated into employment over 100,000 handicapped people in the previous year—another milestone in the growth picture of the public program. To honor the disabled men and women who had achieved rehabilitation, the President also welcomed Edward A. Friskie of Pennsylvania, his wife and three-year-old son Michael, along with Louis Visceri, a Regional Administrator of the Pennsylvania Bureau of Rehabilitation who had been Friskie's counselor earlier. Friskie had been involved in a near-fatal accident which left him with multiple fractures and other injuries so severe that there was little hope he would ever walk or work again. Yet after extensive surgical and rehabilitative procedures, he learned to walk again, first with crutches, then a cane, went back to school and finished college, and at the time of the Washington ceremony, was a successful high school teacher.

The President, facing a barrage of television cameras, radio microphones and wire service photographers, paid tribute to the thousands of people in public and private agencies who made the past year's record possible. But he had formidable competition from little Michael Friskie who scampered about the lawn knocking over microphones, tugging at the President's pants legs and generally launching his own youth movement.

For a select group of people, the summer of 1961 was

saddened by the death in July of John M. Price. If you were an average reader of newspapers, you probably didn't know of it. But if you were a paraplegic or quadriplegic, or close to the rehabilitation work in spinal cord injury, you knew. John Price, a quadriplegic, had created the *Paraplegia News* for the Paralyzed Veterans of America and the National Paraplegia Foundation but his activities ranged far beyond the publication until he became, for thousands of paraplegics, the embodiment of an individual's mastery over the disability. As the *Paraplegia News* said in its tribute to him that fall, ". . . John dedicated every waking hour to the betterment of mankind, wheelchair bound or not . . . He crowded more into his eighteen years as a quadriplegic than most people do in their normal lifetimes . . ."

Of all man's dreams come true, probably nothing quite matched his venture into space. To fly was one phase of the dream, giving man a parity with the winged creatures, yet it represented an extension of man's mastery over the earth. But in May of 1962 Commander Alan B. Shepard, Jr., making the first suborbital flight in his Mercury capsule, and Colonel John H. Glenn, Jr. the following year in man's first orbit of the earth in Friendship 7, were literally reaching for the stars. The future home of mankind would be more than the earth; it would be wherever science could take the species in the universe.

In 1964 there were changes in the leadership of the President's Committee on Employment of the Handicapped. Much-loved General Melvin T. Maas, after ten years as Chairman, died in April. He was succeeded by Harold Russell, now far beyond the days of "The Best Years of Our Lives" and widely known as past National Commander of AMVETS and for his many other achievements.

Appointed as the new Vice Chairman was Dr. Leonard W. Mayo, whose career had embraced exceptional responsibilities as Director of the Association for the Aid of Crippled Children, Chairman of the President's Panel on Mental Retardation, Dean of the School of Applied Social Sciences at Western Reserve University and in other key posts. Continuing as Vice Chairmen were Gordon M. Freeman, Kenneth N. Watson and Victor Riesel.

The rehabilitation research program added another measure of scientific maturity in 1962 with the establishment of the first Research and Training Centers at New York University and the University of Minnesota. In keeping with other research thinking, the new centers were based on the conviction that the broad resources of a major university medical center, linked with a leading clinical facility, could produce advanced rehabilitation research, a strong teaching program to produce well-equipped personnel, and a center of excellence in patient care. Many minds contributed to the R and T Center planning. In the VRA, it was mainly Mary Switzer and Dr. James Garrett. On Capitol Hill Senator Lister Hill and Congressman John Fogarty added their own ideas and their support.

At New York, under Dr. Howard A. Rusk, the Center combined the research capabilities of the Institute of Physical Medicine and Rehabilitation with the New York University Medical Center. In Minneapolis, under Dr. Frederic Kottke and Dr. Frank H. Krusen, the R&T Center brought together the resources of the Kenney Rehabilitation Institute and the University of Minnesota Medical Center. With the initial success of these, the Research and Training Center concept was gradually extended over the next few years to provide such a facility in all major sections of the country: at Baylor University and the Texas Institute for Rehabilitation and Research, under Dr. William A. Spencer; at the University of Washington under Dr. Justus F. Lehmann; at Emory University in Atlanta under Dr. Arthur P. Richardson and Dr. Mieczyslaw Peszcynski; at Tufts University in Massachusetts under Dr. Harold M. Sterling; at Temple University in Pennsylvania under Dr. Frank H. Krusen, who left Minneapolis to return to his alma mater; at George Washington University in Washington, D. C. under Dr. Thomas McP. Brown and Dr. Charles S. Wise; at the University of Colorado under Dr. Jerome W. Gersten; at the University of Southern California under Dr. Austin B. Chin; at the University of Alabama under Dr. William C. Flemming; and at Northwestern University under Dr. Henry B. Betts.

By the mid-sixties, as experience accumulated, the concept of the university-related center was extended beyond medicine to other special fields in rehabilitation. Rehabilitation research and training centers specializing in mental retardation were established at the University of Wisconsin under Dr. F. Rick Heber; at the University of Texas under Dr. William Wolfe; and at the University of Oregon under Dr. Herbert J. Prehm. Specializing in problems peculiar to vocational rehabilitation were the R and T Centers at the University of Arkansas under Dr. Gerald H. Fisher; at the University of Pittsburgh under Dr. Frederick A. Whitehouse; and at the University of West Virginia under one of the early and best-known state directors, F. Ray Power. One center was created to conduct studies and related work in the field of deafness, under Dr. Edna Levine at New York University.

Much the same thinking went into the creation of a network of university-related Regional Research Institutes, designed to provide a laboratory in which the program and operating problems identified by the state vocational rehabilitation agencies could be analyzed, and improved methods developed for solving such problems.

One of the major rehabilitation events of the 1960's

had an odd beginning. In 1963, Crayton Walker, Executive Director of the American Hearing Society (later to become the National Association of Hearing and Speech Agencies) and Mary Switzer, serving a second term as President of the Society, arranged a press conference in Miss Switzer's office as part of the annual observance of National Hearing Week. Present to meet the press were stage and movie star Joan Fontaine and Congressman John Fogarty of Rhode Island. When the briefing and questioning were finished and the press had gone, the principals relaxed and sat about talking. Congressman Fogarty noted that much recent progress had been made on a categorical basis (such as deafness and hearing loss) but he wondered if it might not be time for another organized review of the rehabilitation program broadly, to see where it was, what was going well and what was not, and what ought to be done to assure good programs and growth. He recalled that it had been several years since a study was made (going back to the Task Force on the Handicapped in 1951–1952). Miss Switzer and the others agreed that this would be worthwhile and should be done. She relayed this to Secretary Celebrezze soon after and some preliminary ideas were developed.

Then followed one of those series of fiscal, legislative and administrative misadventures which strains the credulity and patience. The funds and authorization for such a study were not included in the budget. Next time around, when Secretary Celebrezze testified before Mr. Fogarty's appropriations subcommittee, the Secretary was questioned about the study and he assured the Chairman that provisions would be made for it. They were—but by the time this particular shuttlecock had been batted back and forth across the executive-legislative net for the final time and the study group was named, it was 1966. By then a new Secretary, John W. Gardner, had the privilege of appointing the new advisory body for the study—the National Citizens Advisory Committee on Vocational Rehabilitation. And still another Secretary, Wilbur J. Cohen, would receive the Committee's report in June of 1968.

So as it worked out, the man who was responsible for originating the committee never saw the report, nor did he see the 1969 National Conference on Rehabilitation of the Disabled and Disadvantaged which grew out of the Committee's work. Congressman Fogarty died on the day Congress convened in January, 1967.

His death was a serious loss to the nation's public and private rehabilitation programs, for the influence of Mr. Fogarty worked in many and sometimes wondrous ways. He demanded that Federal rehabilitation officials appearing before his appropriation subcommittee give a good accounting for their programs and a solid defense of the funds they were asking. On this, he could be tough. But he also was expert at asking the right sort of questions to lay the written groundwork for the money they needed—and he was basically convinced that rehabilitation programs needed more money.

As a Democrat, Fogarty enjoyed a running feud-of-sorts with the Republican Governor of Rhode Island, John H. Chafee, over whether the vocational rehabilitation program there was developing fast enough. To the extent that any political feuding is good clean fun, this was—good because it was helping the Rhode Island program, clean because it attracted frequent press attention in Rhode Island without demeaning either contestant.

As one of the Hill-Fogarty-Lasker triumvirate, Fogarty was a pivotal man in one of the most remarkable health and rehabilitation sagas of the twentieth century. It had begun in the late Forties, sparked in part by the post-war need for more hospitals, particularly in small towns and rural areas, which led to enactment of the Hill-Burton Hospital Survey and Construction Act.

From this point on, Democratic Senator Lister Hill of Alabama increasingly became the figure and the force behind Federal health legislation and funds. His deep concern with illness, injury, disability and rehabilitation was a natural inheritance; his physician father had named him for the famed English surgeon, Joseph Lister, and many of his close relatives had entered the medical profession. But in choosing law and politics, Senator Hill unquestionably put a far deeper imprint on the history of American medicine than he might if he had followed his father's career.

During his long tenure in the Congress (which totalled, on his retirement at the end of 1968, forty-five years in the House and Senate) he presided for many years over the two key Senate functions in health and rehabilitation—the legislative committee controlling most of the laws, and the appropriations subcommittee controlling nearly all of the money.

Mrs. Mary Lasker, wife of wealthy advertising pioneer Albert Lasker, had set forth on her own crusade for better health and many of her aims converged with those of Senator Hill and Congressman Fogarty. Back in 1942 she and her husband had established the Albert and Mary Lasker Foundation as a financial and operational base for promoting a variety of medical research goals. They had an early and lasting concern for doing something about mental illness, notably about the deplorable conditions in most of the state mental hospitals, but their interests ranged across most of the conditions that threaten mankind, placing a monumental trust in the potential of research—and specifically the research operations of the National Institutes of Health—to find answers to the killing and crippling diseases. When Mr. Lasker died of cancer in 1952, the Foundation's work was firmly established and the "Lasker Operation" was a familiar part of the Washington scene in health and rehabilitation. By the late 1960's, the most obvious monument to the Hill-Fogarty-Lasker labors was the National Institutes of Health, which in some twenty-five years had seen its Federal funds grow to more than a billion dollars annually.

Within the operation, Dr. Rusk served as the key rehabilitation figure, channeling to the rehabilitation research and training programs, the Federal-state vocational rehabilitation program, and the cooperating private programs the momentum of a rising tide of Congressional interest. Closely associated was Mary Switzer who, from her vantage point in the Federal agency, added vigorous program leadership, her own brand of political skill, and the strength of a set of Federal and state programs which obviously were performing together as a "taut ship."

Largely from such an operation, and the Congressional climate it produced, Federal funds for rehabilitation rose steadily during the 1950's and 1960's. More importantly, the funds brought the kinds of results the Congress and other people expected: An increase in the numbers of disabled restored through the Federal-state program, from 58,000 in 1955 to more than 241,000 in 1969, and an increase in research projects into disability and rehabilitation problems, from eighteen in the first year of 1955 to some three hundred in 1969 plus the work of nineteen special Rehabilitation Research and Training Centers and a chain of Regional Research Institutes.

The Hill-Fogarty-Lasker combine, in lending its efforts to the promotion of rehabilitation, was not rowing upstream against a strong current.

In fact, as things function in Washington, two Democrats and a lobbyist cannot, by themselves, accomplish anything. The issue—a much better break for the nation's disabled—was seldom opposed by anyone. The task they performed so brilliantly was to overcome the vague disinterest, the well-intentioned inaction, and the competition from the endless series of crises which constantly preoccupy the minds of official Washington.

There were many to help, from both sides of the political aisle, simply because they believed in the essential principle of restoring the disabled to a useful and self-respecting place in life, and because they had confidence in both the public and private programs.

In the Senate, Republican Senator Norris Cotton of New Hampshire not only believed in the rehabilitation programs but put to work his many years in state and national government to see that they performed efficiently and prospered financially. His fellow Republican Senator Jacob Javits of New York was a constant champion of rehabilitation legislation and funds. Many Democratic Senators, with their party in control of Congress for all but two of the years after World War II, gave the thrust of their leadership to the advancement of rehabilitation, often led by Senator Jennings Randolph of West Virginia, whose long involvement in the problems of the disabled gave him an unofficial deanship in rehabilitation. One of the most vocal and consistently effective champions of the work was Senator Hubert H. Humphrey, whose strong interest continued when he became Vice President. From the time Senator Edward M. Kennedy of Massachusetts entered the Senate in 1962, he gave his personal and sustained efforts to improving and expanding rehabilitation programs both through legislation and funds. Texas Senator Ralph Yarborough was unfailing in his advocacy of the rehabilitation programs and his strength was even more evident when he assumed the chairmanship of the Senate Committee on Labor and Public Welfare following the retirement of Senator Hill in 1968.

In the House, the active interest and support also ranged freely across party lines. From his early experiences with vocational rehabilitation programs, Congressman Carl Perkins of Kentucky developed a sustained interest which was shared by several of his fellow Democrats, notably Hugh L. Carey of New York, Daniel Flood of Pennsylvania, Carleton Sickles of Maryland, Edith Green of Oregon, Dominick V. Daniels of New Jersey and John Brademas of Indiana, and by Republican Congressmen Albert Quie of Minnesota and Ogden R. Reid of New York.

Many professional and voluntary organizations played prominent roles in the growth picture in those years. The National Rehabilitation Association, growing in size and strength with the whole movement, presented the case for rehabilitation legislation and funds persuasively, through such spokesmen as E. B. Whitten, A. P. "Polk" Jarrell of Georgia, Don Russell of Arkansas (and later Commissioner of the Department of Rehabilitation in Virginia), F. Ray Power of West Virginia, O. F. "Freddy" Wise of Alabama, Seid Hendrix of Louisiana and many others.

Goodwill Industries of America, itself growing through the formation of many new Goodwill locals and through increasing stress on rehabilitation, sent its Executive Vice President, P. J. Trevethan and its General Counsel and Legislative Director John C. Harmon, Jr. to Capitol Hill regularly to advise the Congressional committees on legislation which would strengthen and improve the nation's workshops.

Other organizations such as the National Society for Crippled Children and Adults, the Association of Rehabilitation Centers, the American Rehabilitation Foundation, United Cerebral Palsy Associations, National Association of Sheltered Workshops and Homebound Programs helped convey to the committees the needs, the methods and the benefits of rehabilitation programs.

In the early 1960's, several efforts were made to secure changes in the Federal rehabilitation law to meet some obvious needs of both the public and private programs. A number of hearings were held before Congresswoman Edith Green's Special Education Subcommittee but no bill ever reached the House floor. Mrs. Green was in agreement with most of the proposals in the Administration and other bills but she had some ideas of her own, mostly dealing with the financing for the Federal-state program, which she wished to pursue.

In November of 1963, just about everything in Washington—and throughout most of the world—stopped when word came of the senseless assassination of President Kennedy in Texas. Washington is accustomed to pausing at the death of a notable figure but this was no ordinary pause. The shock waves kept coming, a mixture of disbelief and personal agony that arose from millions of people. Before the decade was over, two more figures familiar to those millions would become the victims of the same sort of twisted minds and the nation would mourn the deaths of Senator Robert F. Kennedy and Dr. Martin Luther King. The Decade of the Sixties, begun with such enthusiasm and promise, was becoming the decade of destruction and despair.

There was more than political assassination in the air. An affluent society was being rejected by increasing numbers of young people who found no pleasure, no challenge in the facts or the artifacts of affluence. Black people, moving beyond the 1954 Supreme Court decision striking down the "separate but equal" doctrine in education, were demanding an equal part in all phases of political, social and economic life. Chicanos, American Indians and others were beginning to join in the civil rights movement. Sargent Shriver and his Office of Economic Opportunity were trying to fashion special Federal assistance programs that would direct money and encouragement into new ways of reducing poverty. The increasing involvement in the Vietnam conflict was more than a policy division in government; the public was being involved more deeply in the war as a national issue and the university campuses were becoming forums for resistance and struggle.

In such a rising tide of contention, the ability of the rehabilitation field to retain public interest and support was a tribute to the leadership, in private life and in government. Important things were happening in rehabilitation to help capture this interest. One example was the arrival in the United States in 1964 of Dr. Marian Weiss, Polish surgeon and rehabilitation specialist, for his first "full dress" report on his remarkable research in immediate post-operative fitting of prostheses for amputees. In Poland, amputees were not simply a part of the problem of disability. World War II had left Poland with a fantastic number of amputees, far more than other countries—so many that at one point, amputees were moved out of the cities to avoid an adverse public spectacle. Dr. Rusk had returned from his consultations in Poland in the early 1950's in awe of the enormity of the human damage.

The normal process everywhere in surgical amputations was for the surgery to be done, followed by a waiting period for healing, followed by preliminary fitting of a limb, followed by adjustments and a final limb, followed by training in use of the limb—all of this covering many months (and for many patients, never being completed at all).

Dr. Weiss, head of surgery and rehabilitation at a large rehabilitation hospital outside Warsaw, believed this extended procedure could be drastically shortened. From his research, supported by the international rehabilitation research program of the Vocational Rehabilitation Administration, he had developed a method which permitted the fitting of a temporary prosthesis while the patient was still under anesthesia. When the patient recovered consciousness, the temporary limb was in place; within a few hours the patient could tolerate short periods of weight-bearing. The technique was not feasible for all patients, nor was it the total answer to amputations. Yet it did signal a real breakthrough for large numbers of amputations. The reduction in time lost was dramatic, along with the assurance that surgery and rehabilitation would be one continuous, uninterrupted process. Some of the most valuable results were in the psychological aspects, with most patients avoiding the depression, withdrawal and occasional "phantom pain" experienced in more orthodox procedures.

Although Dr. Weiss' visit was primarily to consult with U. S. surgeons and others, and encourage further studies in this country, his itinerary began with a reception and lecture in Washington sponsored by the Polish Ambassador. The lay guests—from the embassies, State Department and other Washington agencies—were not entirely prepared for Dr. Weiss' color film of his work, particularly the details of the surgery. The ambassador from one of the Eastern European countries fainted.

Another physician, physiatrist William A. Spencer, was honored in Washington that year by the President's Committee on Employment of the Handicapped as its Physician of the Year. The award recognized the exceptional work done by Dr. Spencer in developing and expanding the Texas Institute for Rehabilitation and Research, as a part of the Texas Medical Center at Houston. As one of the early Rehabilitation Research and Training Centers, the Institute had brought to the southwest area a resource for advanced research and teaching as well as a much-needed place for coping with the most difficult and complex problems in severe disability. Emphasizing research in clinical management of patients, the Institute's Dr. Carlos Valbona at that time was pioneering in the development of automated bed-side monitoring systems for the management of critically ill patients, and Dr. Lewis A. Levitt was laying the groundwork for his later studies in the scientific analysis of gait patterns among lower limb amputees and others with ambulation problems.

By early 1965 the wheels were turning again to make changes in the Federal rehabilitation law. It had been eleven years since the last major revisions and a variety of improve-ments in the Federal machinery was needed. Meetings and discussions had been held with many organizations and the general type of legislation needed was largely agreed upon, so that there was no major opposition to the legislation sent to Congress by President Lyndon B. Johnson and Secretary Celebrezze.

The bills moved through House and Senate hearings and by July of 1965 cleared the House. There was a summer hiatus, caused mostly by a log jam of other legislation in the Senate, which held up the bill but it finally passed the Senate on October 1 and was signed by President Johnson at his Texas White House on November 8. The fifth legislative benchmark in the long history of the public rehabilitation program had been carved.

The new Act changed the financing system for the Federal-state program of vocational rehabilitation, increas-ing the Federal share of costs to seventy-five percent and specifying in the basic law the amounts to be allotted an-nually among the states. A program of construction assis-tance was authorized, to build more rehabilitation centers and workshops, and to expand present ones, along with as-sistance in initial staffing costs. A new set of grant programs was inaugurated to help improve workshops for the handi-capped, including a system for paying handicapped trainees a modest allowance while undergoing training. A National Policy and Performance Council was established, through which non-government experts could help frame policy on workshop improvement and maintain a regular review of progress. Funds were authorized for a national effort in state-wide planning, encouraging each state to assess its rehabilitation resources and draw plans for putting new facilities and services in localities where they were needed most. A National Commission on Architectural Barriers was created to take advantage of the early work done by such organizations as the National Society for Crippled Children Children and Adults and the President's Committee on Employment of the Handicapped, to make buildings more accessible to people in wheelchairs, on braces and crutches, and otherwise limited in their locomotion. The training program for preparing more professional and technical workers in rehabilitation was broadened to clearly authorize up to four years of aid for students and to specify the fields of work for which training assistance could be furnished.

The main reason for the delay in the rehabilitation bill that summer was the heavy preoccupation of the Congress, and particularly the Senate, with the Medicare amendments to the Social Security Act. Probably nothing before the Congress for several years had generated such intense political controversy. The idea of a national system of health care for older people was at least as old as the Social Security Act itself. Legislation to provide for such a program, in one form or another, had been before the Congress for more than twenty years. All those years of conflicting views, of heated and often bitter debate, came to a boil in the Senate in August of 1965. Marathon bargaining sessions, rearranged strategy, compromises and revisions—all left their birthmark on the bill that emerged from the Senate. In the long, final days, only a few people seemed to even know what had happened at the end of the day. One of these was HEW Under Secretary Wilbur Cohen, master planner in Social Security for thirty years and the Administration's spokesman and strategist in the battle for Medicare.

It was remarkable that, in all the swirling events, he remembered to see that an important rehabilitation provision stayed in the bill. For two years there had been agreement in the Department, between Social Security Commissioner Robert Ball and VRA Commissioner Mary Switzer that Social Security Trust Funds should be used to pay for vocational rehabilitation services for disability beneficiaries of the Social Security program who could be restored to activity and work. Mr. Cohen saw to it that this was included in the same bill which launched the Medicare program.

One of the many unfortunate facets of the compromise Medicare law was the fact that it was constructed as a predominantly acute care program rather than a complete care program for the aged. Along with subsequent amendments, Medicare accepted the idea of extended care facilities and home care programs, not because they were always the best places to provide the care needed but because they seemed cheaper. Combined with pressures to empty hospital beds as fast as possible, the Medicare program had the effect of discouraging rehabilitation for older patients who were the victims of severe injuries or illnesses.

In the "Medicare month" of August, 1965, John W. Gardner was named Secretary of Health, Education and Welfare. All new Secretaries inherit a large package of someone else's thinking but Mr. Gardner's inheritance was larger than most. In addition to Medicare, there was the ballooning push in Federal aid to education, the annual contest for an appropriation bill which was not of his making, an unpopular welfare program made even less palatable by the large-scale projects of Sargent Shriver's OEO poverty program, and the largest legislative program in the history of HEW.

Yet he took time for a long luncheon session with Mary Switzer and her top staff, to familiarize himself with the vocational rehabilitation program and to help make sure that the 1965 amendments to the Act, still pending in the Senate, would not be lost.

He had other close sources besides Commissioner Switzer and Under Secretary Cohen for weighing the worth of the rehabilitation programs. The Assistant Secretary and Comptroller, James F. Kelly and his Deputy for budget, James B. Cardwell, lived with the schizophrenic problem of fighting off Departmental budget increases from within while defending the budget to the death from the outside. Kelly put the rehabilitation budget requests through his expert wringer. But basically he believed that the vocational rehabilitation programs represented one of the best investments the government made in people, and the budgets he and Cardwell took before the Department's Budget Committee and the Bureau of the Budget reflected this.

So with a greatly broadened new Federal law in November of 1965 and with strong budget support, the rehabilitation programs faced the last half of the Sixties with enthusiasm, confidence and the feeling that before long, this country could actually bring under control the vast problem of disability among the American people.

CHAPTER VIII

THE VIEW FROM
A NEW PLATEAU

———◆◆◆◆————

THE LAST HALF of the 1960's was a mélange of achievement, disenchantment, progress, violence, discovery and division. The buffeting of social, legal and industrial institutions did not leave the rehabilitation field untouched, yet the basic stability of its programs was never jeopardized. As an individualized restorative effort, as an avenue to jobs and income for those least able to compete in the marketplace, public and private programs of rehabilitation continued, for the most part, outside the public clamor and off the television screens.

On the international scene, Eugene J. Taylor was honored with the Lasker Award, along with three other leaders from foreign countries, at the Tenth World Congress of the International Society for Rehabilitation of the Disabled in Wiesbaden, Germany in 1966. At that meeting the International Society bade farewell to its long-time Secretary General, Donald V. Wilson, who was assuming the Presidency of the Leonard Wood Memorial for the Eradication of Leprosy, and later to be Deputy to the National Director of Goodwill Industries of America, Robert E. Watkins. The reins were taken over for several months by Dorothy Warms who had served the Society so ably for many years. The final choice for a new Secretary General was Norman Acton, long a leader in international work and thoroughly versed in rehabilitation programs for the disabled.

The following year a National Theatre of the Deaf was created as a professional touring company. It was the outgrowth of the ideas of Anne Bancroft, who earlier had scored so brilliantly in her Academy Award–winning "The Miracle Worker," and her director Arthur Penn. Both had been deeply impressed when they saw a performance of "Othello" by deaf players at Gallaudet College in Washington. With the enthusiastic support of Mary Switzer and Boyce Williams, a career leader in work for the deaf at the VRA, the repertory group was formed and within two years had proved that such a touring company could not only produce vivid theatre but could survive the commercial problems of the theatrical world.

By 1967 the rehabilitation center established by Dr. Paul Magnuson in Chicago thirteen years before had become a victim of the rehabilitation trend: the waiting list of disabled patients seeking admission to the Rehabilitation Institute of Chicago was too long, the Institute building was too small and too ancient. The excellence of the Institute's work, under Dr. Magnuson, his fellow orthopedist and long-time close associate Dr. Clinton L. Compere, and Dr. Henry Betts, the Medical Director, was well known. It was, in fact, this excellence which accounted for the waiting list, and had caused the Vocational Rehabilitation Administration in Washington to consider designating the facility as a Rehabilitation Research and Training Center to serve that section of the Midwest.

A hard decision, involving large amounts of money and calling for a vast amount of community support, had to be made, and it was: to build a new high-rise Institute, as a part of the Northwestern University Medical Center complex, to provide quarters for research, teaching, expanded patient care, for the Prosthetics Research Center of Northwestern, and for an enlarged school of physical therapy.

A major factor in the decision to proceed was the fact that James O. Heyworth, successful Chicago businessman and supporter of the Institute, agreed to give up his business career and head the Institute's new organization, with particular responsibilities for construction of the new building.

Dr. Magnuson did not live to see the final plans for the new Institute. He died in November of 1969. But he would have a proper memorial in the new building, a testament to an energetic, creative orthopedist who found in rehabilitation of the disabled a sustained satisfaction that he could not quite find in surgery alone.

The Vocational Rehabilitation Act was amended again in 1967 to meet several specialized needs, including separate provisions for the rehabilitation of much-neglected migratory workers and to eliminate residence requirements for disabled people needing rehabilitation services. But the outstanding feature of the new changes was the authorization to construct and operate a National Center for Deaf-Blind Youths and Adults. For decades before her death, Helen Keller had dreamed of and worked for such an institution, a place where the victims of this overwhelming calamity could find the highly specialized, devoted people they must have in order to establish a link with the rest of the world and make places for themselves in the human community. Many people had shared her dream but it was Peter Salmon, Director of the Industrial Home for the Blind in New York, and the dean of the nation's workers in the field of blindness and deaf-blindness, who provided the determined leadership to make the dream come true. Exhibit A in the long effort for the Center was his associate Robert J. Smithdas, himself deaf and blind, whose attainments in education and executive leadership had earned for him the "Handicapped American of the Year" in 1965 from the President's Committee on Employment of the Handicapped. The Federal action enabled the Center to begin promptly in temporary quarters on Long Island and by 1970, with Federal funds available and a site selected at Sands Point, L. I., construction of the new, permanent Center was assured.

In the same period, the Congress provided for the Bureau of Education for the Handicapped in the U. S. Office of Education to finance a series of regionally-distributed centers to serve deaf-blind children. Under the leadership of Dr. Edward Martin, Associate Commissioner of Education and head of the Bureau, who had supervised the tremendous expansion of education programs for handicapped children, most of the children's centers were in operation by the end of the 1960's.

In the summer of 1967 the Department of HEW made some drastic organizational changes involving the rehabilitation agency. As the pressing problems of the poor and the racial minorities demanded more and more attention everywhere, the Department struggled with ways to realign its organizations to do a better job of solving these problems. A major step was the creation of the Social and Rehabilitation Service, designed to bring together in a better way the service-giving and support programs and to emphasize rehabilitation. The welfare functions were separated into a welfare payments agency, a medical service agency to administer the Medicaid program, and a welfare service group. The Administration on Aging was made a part of the new SRS, as was the juvenile delinquency agency.

The vocational rehabilitation agency, renamed the Rehabilitation Services Administration, also became a bureau of the new SRS. Out of its long and successful experience in restoring disabled people to useful lives, the RSA was seen as an organization which could transfer its concepts and methods to the problems and needs of the disadvantaged generally. Named Commissioner of the new RSA was Joseph Hunt, who for so many years had been a key executive in the rehabilitation agency.

Mary Switzer, from her post as long-time head of the rehabilitation agency, was appointed the first Administrator of the Social and Rehabilitation Service. Dr. James F. Garrett became the Assistant Administrator in charge of SRS research and professional training.

In March of the next year, following the departure of Secretary Gardner, Under Secretary Wilbur J. Cohen was nominated (and quickly confirmed by the Senate) as Secretary of Health, Education and Welfare. It climaxed a long career, begun as a staff member of the Social Security Board in the 1930's, and covering most of the crucial times in the history of the Federal Security Agency and HEW.

The place of rehabilitation centers and workshops in the rehabilitation field was formalized in 1968 with the establishment of the Commission on Accreditation of Rehabilitation Facilities. The long years of work by so many Center Directors and workshop administrators, to create a level of standards which would give the rehabilitation professionals, the public and disabled people a strong sense of confidence in the specialized services of rehabilitation facilities, had borne fruit.

Named to direct the new accreditation system was Charles Caniff who had given many years of devoted work to the National Paraplegia Foundation, to the elimination of architectural barriers faced by handicapped people, and to facility improvement. The Commission was aided by the Joint Commission on Accreditation of Hospitals and drew heavily on its experience.

In July of that year, another set of specialized amendments to the Vocational Rehabilitation Act was passed by the Congress, marking the third time the law had been revised in four years. Of the changes, two were of primary significance. One was an increase in the Federal share of the basic Federal-state program costs from seventy-five percent to eighty percent (from three Federal dollars to four for each dollar of state funds). The other was to authorize a new and separate grant program of vocational evaluation and work adjustment, which would place the state agencies in a position to function as the central points for seeing virtually all handicapped people with problems requiring special help, providing services to those who were eligible for vocational rehabilitation assistance, and placing others in the hands of appropriate community agencies. (The Congress subsequently declined to fund this new program, so that its possibilities had not been tested as the program moved into the Seventies.)

There were other changes—to formally incorporate into the law the "Laird Amendment" which technically had been in force for several years; to authorize contracts with industry for training handicapped people; and to establish "New Careers" programs to help handicapped people secure training and jobs in rehabilitation work and in a variety of kinds of public service employment.

In the fall of 1968 a new organization was formed in the health education field. The Association of Schools of Allied Health Professions was the brainchild of Dr. Darrel J. Mase, long active in rehabilitation affairs and in health manpower, who years before had established the first college program for training a variety of related personnel under one organizational structure in the College of Health Related Professions at the J. Hillis Miller Health Center, University of Florida at Gainesville. As the idea of such integrated administration and teaching slowly spread to other teaching institutions, Dr. Mase became convinced that a national organization for joint planning and problem-solving was needed. He was joined by Dr. J. Warren Perry, Dean of the School of Health Related Professions at the State University of New York at Buffalo, who had directed prosthetics research at Northwestern University and the Rehabilitation Institute of Chicago, and subsequently served as Deputy Assistant Commissioner for Research and Training in the Vocational Rehabilitation Administration in HEW. With heavy financial support and encouragement from the W. K. Kellog Foundation, the Association established headquarters in Washington and began a program of cooperative planning, research and recruitment to advance allied health training.

In November of 1968 the voters elected a new Republican President, Richard M. Nixon over the Democratic nominee, Hubert H. Humphrey. Vice President Humphrey made a race of it in the popular vote, with Mr. Nixon winning by only about 500,000 out of some 72,000,000 votes cast, but in the electoral vote, the President-elect won handily. For the new President, it was the peak of a long career in public office—as a Congressman, Senator and as Vice President in the Eisenhower Administration.

Named Secretary of HEW in the new Administration was Robert W. Finch, former Lieutenant Governor of California and active in the direction of the 1968 campaign.

California was doing more than sending a successful Presidential candidate to the White House. The Federal-state program of vocational rehabilitation was continuing to grow into one of the largest in the nation, as befitted a state with such a soaring population. In Los Angeles, the County Board of Supervisors signed a contract in late 1968 affiliating Rancho Los Amigos Hospital with the University of Southern California School of Medicine, giving the chronic disease and rehabilitation programs of Rancho the added benefits of a major medical school, its faculty and resources, and providing the school with a stimulating new teaching hospital.

The end of the Sixties was a time for fiftieth anniversaries for those many organizations which had been born in the beginnings of twentieth century rehabilitation. In 1967 the American Occupational Therapy Association observed its beginnings fifty years before. Four of the Association's former Presidents—Ruth W. Brunyate, Colonel Ruth A. Robinson, Wilma L. West and Helen Willard— pooled their wide experience in the profession to provide an absorbing account of OT's origins and its development into an integral part of the health and rehabilitation picture in the United States.

At the Institute for the Crippled and Disabled, now under the skillful direction of Dr. Salvatore G. DiMichael, a year-long series of special events, movies and publications told the story of the historic work done there fifty years before and in the intervening years. To honor the founder, the Board of Trustees presented a special scroll to Jeremiah Milbank "on behalf of all those who lives have been enriched by his work." The commencement address for 202 handicapped people completing their rehabilitation program was given by Bob Hope, who toured the Institute and said, "I feel a lot taller for what I have seen here today."

The following year the Institute opened its new research facility, the Milbank Research Laboratories, providing a new avenue for investigation into spinal cord injury and other disabling conditions, and leading to a new mission and a new name for the pioneer center, the ICD Rehabilitation and Research Center.

In 1969 the National Easter Seal Society for Crippled

Children and Adults looked back to Elyria, Ohio and its founding fifty years before. An important part of their anniversary celebrations was the recognition of the Rotary Clubs of America for the early and sustained support they had given to the National Society's rehabilitation work for crippled children. A glimpse of what had been happening was provided by their fund raising figures: in the first year of Easter Seal sales in 1934, they had raised $47,052. In 1967 the total was more than $16 million.

Those state rehabilitation agencies whose roots went back to the days of World War I held a series of anniversaries, beginning with Massachusetts in 1968. The next year there were eight more celebrations. New Jersey honored its pioneers including Dr. Albee and Colonel Bryant and its recently-retired Director, Mrs. Beatrice Holderman. In a special tribute, Dr. Henry Kessler, himself the architect of much of New Jersey's progress over nearly five decades, presented the Golden Jubilee Award of the New Jersey Rehabilitation Commission to Jeremiah Milbank for his pioneering role in fostering the state's first rehabilitation law.

In Rhode Island, where the vocational rehabilitation program commemorated its fiftieth year in 1969, the contrast between the beginnings and the present was particularly sharp. In the first decade, when the original Director, Dr. Charles Carroll, was nurturing a small program in a small state, a ten-year total of 152 disabled people was served. In the one year of 1969, when another Director, thirty-year veteran George F. Moore, Jr. was presiding over one of the most aggressive programs in the nation, 9,919 disabled were served. Obviously the political volleyball back in the early Sixties between Republican Governor Chafee (now Secretary of the Navy in Washington) and Democratic Congressman Fogarty had had some tangible results —a better rehabilitation program for the people of Rhode Island.

In May of 1969 the Curative Workshop of Milwaukee reached its fiftieth milestone of service to the disabled in Wisconsin. The size and character of that service bore little resemblance to what Elizabeth Upham had set in motion so long before; in the 1968 year, the CWM had served over five thousand patients referred to them by more than nine hundred physicians, and their budget that year was well over a million dollars.

Pennsylvania joined the anniversary parade in 1969 with special observances to mark the beginnings and to pay tribute to the state rehabilitation program which for several years had rehabilitated more disabled people annually than any other state (they totalled more than sixteen thousand in 1969). It was also the year when Charles L. Eby, State Director since 1958—a period when the agency experienced some of its greatest growth in services—retired and was succeeded by one of the program's most able administrators, Lee V. Kebach.

Some shock waves went through a lot of rehabilitation workers early in 1969, particularly among those in Washington, when President Nixon nominated Congressman Melvin R. Laird of Wisconsin as the new Secretary of Defense. Rehabilitation fans of "Mel" Laird were delighted with his new Cabinet post, with the honor that went with the new appointment, but they crossed their fingers at the prospect of his loss to the rehabilitation "movement." His selection as the Secretary of Defense obviously was a fine choice, for he had become an expert on military affairs through his long membership on the military appropriations subcommittee. But he also had served for many years as the ranking minority member of the House Appropriations Subcommittee for the Departments of Labor and Health, Education and Welfare—and in that seat had become one of the most widely known Congressional figures in the development of rehabilitation programs. Not everyone knew of his prolonged efforts to clear up the problems of a rehabilitation facility back home in Racine but everyone knew of the "Laird Amendment." Dozens of rehabilitation facilities in every section of the country had been aided by that amendment, which was in itself a bit of legislative legerdemain, effecting a permanent change in law through the appropriation process.

As it worked out, his successor as senior Republican on the appropriations subcommittee was also a person with more than passing interest in, and knowledge about, rehabilitation programs. Congressman Robert Michel of Illinois had taken a strong interest in the requests for rehabilitation funds before the committee and he had gained some first-hand experience with a prominent rehabilitation center back home in Peoria, through the work of Dr. Rex O. McMorris and the Institute of Physical Medicine and Rehabilitation there.

Illinois, in fact, developed something of a rehabilitation contingent. On the other side of Capitol Hill, Senator Charles Percy frequently took a strong hand in rehabilitation affairs, evincing his interest in the Rehabilitation Institute of Chicago, the Illinois vocational rehabilitation program and many other phases of the work. In the House, Congressman Sidney Yates of Chicago became a strong advocate of expanded rehabilitation services for the disabled in his district and elsewhere.

A national conference was convened in Washington in June of 1969 which had a different character from any previous rehabilitation meetings. The National Conference on Rehabilitation of the Disabled and Disadvantaged was one result of the deliberations of the National Citizens Advisory Committee on Vocational Rehabilitation, which had devoted two years of work to extensive studies of public and private rehabilitation programs. Chaired by Dr. Howard A. Rusk, the committee membership was rich in diversity of backgrounds, including W. Scott Allan, Assistant Vice President of Liberty Mutual Insurance Company, a leading figure in Liberty Mutual's active program of rehabilitation, and a Past President of the National Rehabilitation Association; Mrs. John A. Burns who, as wife of the Governor of Hawaii, had demonstrated that a paraplegic in a wheelchair can preside with poise, charm and efficiency over a Governor's Mansion; and Alfred Slicer who, as Director of the Illinois Division of Vocational Rehabilitation, headed one of the largest and most effective programs in the nation.

From private life there was Mrs. Mary Duke Biddle Semans, an active figure in health and rehabilitation development in North Carolina and elsewhere, Chairman of the Mary Duke Biddle Foundation and wife of Dr. James H. Semans, a leading urologist and himself widely known for his work in spinal cord injuries. From organized labor there was Dr. William O. Kuhl, Director of Research and Education for the International Brotherhood of Boilermarkers, Iron Shipbuilders, Blacksmiths, Forgers and Helpers. From industry there was Edgar J. Forio, retired Senior Vice-President of the Coca Cola Company. Dr. Hester Turner, National Director of the Camp Fire Girls and former Dean of Students at Lewis and Clark College in Portland, Oregon brought to the group a wealth of knowledge in the problems of children and youth. From San Francisco, Mrs. Jacqueline M. Smith, member of the city's Social Service Commission, added knowledge of West Coast needs and the realistic social problems of disabled people in urban settings. The special requirements of blind people were ably portrayed within the Committee by Burt L. Risley, one of the country's best-known leaders in rehabilitation work as Executive Director of the Texas State Commission for the Blind.

The report of the Committee was, in itself, a text on the problems of disability and rehabilitation, and of the tremendous potential which existed in this country for converting promise into reality for millions of disabled people. The Committee staff, headed by Richard A. Grant and Dr. Eleanor Poland, had brought into the effort the experience, data and views of dozens of national organizations and informed individuals, through a series of hearings at various points in the country, supplemented by a large volume of inquiries through correspondence and meetings.

One paragraph of the Committee report conveyed the essentials of the case for expanded rehabilitation services for the disabled in the United States: "We are a humane nation and we are a nation of businessmen. Yet we violate the principles of humanity and business when we continue to permit large numbers of Americans to languish in the shadow of a serious handicap which could be mastered. Both the conscience and the purse suffer when men and women who could be self-reliant and productive are consigned to futility and dependency."

From discussions of the report, particularly in light of the aims of the new Social and Rehabilitation Service, there grew plans for a national conference. Assembled at the Mayflower Hotel in Washington in June of 1969, the National Citizens Conference on Rehabilitation of the Disabled and Disadvantaged under the co-chairmanship of W. Scott Allan and Dr. Rusk brought together for the first time a large group of "consumers" and rehabilitation professionals. Militant groups formed among blacks, Chicanos and American Indians, demanding a strong voice in the planning and provision of services, rehabilitation attention to the problems of narcotics addiction and alcoholism, and programs for the public offender. At times the tenor of the conference ranged from raucous to rebellious. Most obvious was the fact that the minority speakers knew little about rehabilitation programs for the disabled and that many of the rehabilitation professionals were having their first direct exposure to the language and lives of minority people.

Along with the person-to-person learning process that was so evident at the conference, there was a new realization that better ways must be developed to find, and establish links with, the thousands of poor people, both among the white and minority groups, who were living outside the mainstream of rehabilitation development. Working with disabled people in poverty circumstances was not new in rehabilitation; it was as old as the rehabilitation concept itself. But the rehabilitation fraternity was finding what a whole society was finding—that within the structure of American life, social islands exist which seldom have been reached in the workings of "the system." In the long growth of rehabilitation programs, far too few of the disabled people in these clusters of isolation had even been aware that such programs existed.

As the end of the decade neared, many changes were apparent in the faces and the places which constituted the image of rehabilitation in the United States. At Adelphi University on Long Island, Dr. June S. Rothberg was named the new Dean of the School of Nursing, placing one of rehabilitation nursing's leading figures in a place of prominence in nursing education. Dr. Rothberg, as Principal Investigator, had conducted a nursing rehabilitation study project back in the late 1950's out of Goldwater Memorial Hospital in New York. She subsequently represented the American Nursing Association with the Commission on Accreditation of Rehabilitation Facilities, became the first nurse to be an active member of the American Congress of Rehabilitation Medicine and gained national prominence as a leader in nursing education.

The Rehabilitation Services Administration in Washington came under a new leader in October of 1969 with the appointment of Dr. Edward Newman as Commissioner. In Massachusetts he had directed statewide studies of rehabilitation needs and of the mental retardation problems of the Commonwealth. Immediately before assuming office he had spent a year with the Federal Bureau of the Budget, which probably is about the best preparatory school a Federal administrator can attend.

One event signalled the end of an era. On December 7, 1969 the weekly column of Dr. Rusk appeared for the last time in *The New York Times*. The date of that last column was curiously tied to the Rusk history, for it was Pearl Harbor on December 7, twenty-eight years before, which had brought Rusk into the military service where he first committed himself to the task of restoring the sick, injured and disabled, and projected him eventually into a world-wide role in the advancement of rehabilitation—and it was December 7, 1945 when the *Times* column had first appeared.

As Rusk pointed out in the final column, the original objective of publisher Arthur Hays Sulzburger—to bring the benefits of rehabilitation to a vastly larger number of Americans—had been achieved.

And yet, the 1970's opened upon a sea of need among disabled people which was, in its own way, as great and demanding as the situation fifty years before. From the 523 disabled rehabilitated back in 1921, the Federal-state program had grown to the point where nearly 267,000 were restored in 1970. Over those years a total of more than 2,500,000 people had been rehabilitated through the public program alone, with additional millions served by the many private organizations.

But what the United States had accomplished was not mastery over the problems of disability but rather the know-how to do it on a wide front. Just as Pasteur and Lister had opened the door of science on medicine without solving the problems of medical care, so had the rehabilitation pioneers produced the technical knowledge to deal effectively with disabling conditions without achieving the size or the operating methods to assert control over them.

The demands for rehabilitation services kept running ahead of the capacity to serve. Part of the demand arose out of a nation that kept growing, from a little under 92,000,000 people in 1900 to more than 200,000,000 in 1970. Part of it came from the simple fact that as rehabilitation acquired more scientific and technical knowledge, it became able to restore far more people, many of whom could not have been helped at all in the earlier years. But other equally potent factors were at work: the national and state governments increasingly built provisions for rehabilitation into new laws, such as Medicare, Medicaid, welfare, workmen's compensation, veterans programs and others, producing requirements upon public and private rehabilitation programs alike; the public was increasing its demands for many things, including rehabilitation services; new drugs and new surgical methods were saving lives in diseases and injuries where formerly there was no hope, and in the process creating new candidates for rehabilitation.

In February of 1970, Mary Switzer retired from her post as Administrator of the Social and Rehabilitation Service, ending one of the most remarkable careers in the Federal service. During her 49 years in government, she had served the nation in many ways but she would be remembered, above all, for using her role in Washington as a vehicle to help both public and private rehabilitation programs move ahead together in the greatest growth period in rehabilitation history. Although she left the Federal service, she did not leave rehabilitation; she was named a Vice President and head of the Washington office of the World Rehabilitation Fund.

Replacing her as Administrator of the Social and Re-habilitation service was John D. Twiname, formerly a top official of the American Hospital Supply Corporation, who had come to the agency a year before as Deputy Adminis-trator.

At the helm of the Department of Health, Education and Welfare there was a new Secretary that year, Elliot L. Richardson of Massachusetts. He came to the post with a knowledge of many of HEW's activities, including the re-habilitation program. As a former Lieutenant Governor and as Attorney General in Massachusetts, he knew state govern-ment. As Secretary and Treasurer of Massachusetts General Hospital and in many other capacities, he knew about the workings of rehabilitation programs at the level of the dis-abled patient. As Assistant Secretary for Legislation in HEW during the Eisenhower Administration, he had learned about the Federal-state program of vocational rehabilitation in the Mary Switzer school of indoctrination. So the Rehabilitation Services Administration would have an informed executive at the top in HEW.

The Federal-state program of vocational rehabilitation had its own fiftieth anniversary that year, observed with cere-monies for Senators, Congressmen and other officials in Washington, and with a series of observances in most of the states to honor the state directors and others who had given distinction and leadership to the program over the years.

In November, in what certainly was the quietest of the ceremonies, President Nixon honored Jeremiah Milbank by awarding to him the gold medallion struck for the obser-vance of the Fiftieth Anniversary of the Federal-state pro-gram. The presentation was made to Jeremiah Milbank, Jr. on behalf of his father, whose health would not permit a trip to Washington. In conferring the honor, the President expressed his gratitude for the pioneering work done so long before by Mr. Milbank, both in establishing the Institute for the Crippled and Disabled in 1917 and in his strong support for passage of the first Federal vocational rehabilitation law. The small group that gathered for the tribute included family members Mrs. H. Lawrence Bogert, who had shared her father's plans and labors at the Institute and still served as Chairman of its Board of Trustees, and Jeremiah Milbank III, a member of the White House staff. There was Herman G. Place of New York, President of the ICD, Col. Frank E. Mason of Leesburg, Virginia, a life-long friend of the elder Mr. Milbank, and Dr. Edward Newman, Commissioner of the Rehabilitation Services Administration in Washington.

And so the Decade of the Seventies was begun with a grateful look back at the Twenties.

There was much to be grateful for, particularly if you were disabled and in need of help.

EPILOGUE

———◄•••►———

IT IS TIME again to take another look at disability in this country, at what can be done to prevent it, at what can be done through rehabilitation to control it.

The characteristics of disabling conditions among the American people, as well as efforts to cope with them, have undergone a steady series of changes during the Twentieth Century. Paraplegia was not a problem seventy years ago, for nearly all its victims died; today paraplegia is a major problem. Tuberculosis was everywhere at the beginning of the century and efforts to control it and restore the tuberculous helped give rehabilitation work its early start; today it is a secondary health and rehabilitation concern. An account of the disabling conditions which have largely disappeared, and of the new forms of disability that have emerged, would be a long one. Adding to the changing workload picture has been the increasing ability of rehabilitation experts to restore many disabled people who previously had no hope of becoming active again.

Rehabilitation programs themselves have changed in size, composition, outreach, cost and their relationship to communities and government. With the number of disabled being rehabilitated through the Federal-state program now approaching 300,000 annually, and with other thousands being restored through the many voluntary programs, the scope of present efforts might seem adequate. But by the most conservative estimates, there are from six million to eight million disabled people who need rehabilitation help. The present combined capacities of public and private programs cannot even keep up with the new cases appearing each year.

Similarly, the striking contrast between the near-vacuum in trained personnel and special facilities which existed at the beginning of the century and the supply in 1970 represents dramatic progress but not victory. The National Rehabilitation Association, for example, now lists nearly 35,000 members, the American Occupational Therapy Association some 12,000, the American Physical Therapy Association about 17,000, the American Speech and Hearing Association 13,000. More than 800 physicians are certified by the American specialty board in Physical Medicine and Rehabilitation. Other professional and technical specialty fields have shown similar growth. Rehabilitation facilities—centers, workshops, special facilities, rehabilitation departments in hospitals and others—now total around 4,000, of which perhaps half are of sufficient size and scope to provide a substantial range of services. (Nearly 1,600 of the workshops have special wage rate certificates from the Department of Labor.)

Despite these gains, there are few rehabilitation centers which do not have a waiting list, few state rehabilitation agencies which do not have to guard against running out of funds each year because they are faced with more requests for service than they can handle promptly.

As the Congress has gained experience over the years

in making use of the public rehabilitation program to help solve a variety of medical and social problems, it has built the Federal-state program into more and more Federal laws. This trend will accelerate in the 1970's and, because state agencies turn to private organizations and groups for most of their service, both public and private agencies will be confronted with larger and larger demands for service, buttressed by law.

Our attitudes and our methods in relation to the causes of disabling impairments are changing. The recent approaches to accident prevention and consumer protection, which are striving to take the hazards out of products before they reach the consumer, may turn out to be one of the most decisive trends ever set in motion with respect to the prevention and control of disabling conditions. It is quite possible to "engineer out" a tremendous amount of human damage and to legislate out still more. If this approach is tenaciously pursued, and if safety education for the individual is continued and improved, millions of Americans can be spared the tragedies of a serious disability.

It is time now for comprehensive medical restorative services to be built into our medical care systems. In trying to get this done, we are in many ways the victims of our own rehabilitation history. For the most part, the medical restoration of the disabled has developed as something additional and optional, as something that hopefully gets done later, after the patient goes home.

There no longer is any excuse for forcing a severely disabled patient to go home and wait for months or years for the medical restorative procedures which could and should have been done—with greater success and less cost —as a part of his initial medical care. There no longer is any excuse for making artificial distinctions between "acute care" and "restorative care," for both are essential to the recovery process. Promptness and continuity of care, along with quality and completeness of service, should govern decisions on where the restorative care is provided, whether in the same hospital, or a medical rehabilitation center, or other specialized rehabilitation facility.

Because the nature and the aims of rehabilitation range well beyond the medical restoration phases, there is a great need to expand and improve the work of vocational rehabilitation centers, workshops and special facilities for the disabled. As a nation, we are trying to honestly confront and bring under control the massive and often-shocking conditions of poverty among millions of Americans. Until we face up to the enormous problems of the most disadvantaged of all—the severely disabled poor—we will never master either disability or poverty in this country. Beyond the widespread need for medical restorative service for these men, women and children, there must be far better provisions for giving them the skills, the work orientation, the job openings and the confidence in themselves they will need to find useful and satisfying places in life.

We now are getting the results of long years of effort to make better provisions for the disabled in many of our regular service programs for people. Special education for the handicapped, for example, which for so many decades was more of a name than a service program, has grown to large proportions and will continue to expand. (Federal funds alone totalled about a quarter billion dollars for 1970–1971.) Manpower training and employment programs have grown solidly and have slowly begun to give more attention and resources to the handicapped. Other specialized supportive programs aiding the disabled in substantial ways have come along.

This clear trend should tell the rehabilitation agencies, both public and private, that it is time to begin concentrating their great expertise on those with the most difficult and demanding disabilities, where no one else can provide a solution. For the most part, rehabilitation agencies have functioned against the background of an extremely flexible set of admission and eligibility rules. These rules should be critically examined and revised to place the specialized competency of the rehabilitation organizations squarely behind the requirements of those who will never "make it" without their help.

Rehabilitation programs have grown and acquired respect because, over the years, they have been able to respond to a variety of changing situations. It is time now to rise to the requirements of still another.

INDEX

Employment Bureau for the Handicapped, 13
Employment Service, 113, 134
Erskine, Gen. Graves B., 102
"Evergreen," 21
Ewing, Oscar, 111

Fairbanks, Douglas, 35
Faries, Dr. John Culbert, 12, 87
Faulkes, W. F., 39, 41, 45, 58
Federal Board for Vocational Education, 15, 16, 17, 18, 24, 25, 32, 37
— Emergency Relief Administration, 56, 57
— Security Agency, 68, 111, 113, 117, 156
Federation of Associations for Cripples, 12
Fernbach, Frank L., 113
Fess, Sen. Simeon D., 34, 44
Finch, Robert W., 158
Fish, Marjorie, 91
Fisher, Dr. Gerald H., 138
Fisk University, 116
Flemming, Arthur S., 112
Flemming, Dr. William C., 138
Flood, Rep. Daniel, 144
Fogarty, Rep. John, 137, 139, 140, 141, 142, 160
Fontaine, Joan, 139
Food Administration, 48
Ford, Henry, 47
Forio, Edgar J., 163
Foster, T. C., 39, 54
Francis, Archduke, 8
Freeman, Gordon M., 137
Friskie, Edward A., Michael, 135

Gallaudet College, 6, 153
Gardner, John W., 139, 150, 156
Garrett, Dr. James, 88, 96, 104, 115, 137, 156
Geiger, Davis B., 113
Gellman, Dr. William, 103
George Washington University, 138; Medical School, 113
Gerber, Dr. Joseph H., 114
German National Federation for the Care of Cripples, 10
Gersten, Dr. Jerome W., 138
Gilbreth, Frank, Frank, Jr., Lillian, 19
Girl Scouts, 113
Gish, Lillian, 35

Glenn, Col. John H., Jr., 136
Goldsthwait, Col. Joel E., 20
Goldwater Memorial Hospital, 165
Goodman, Benny, 66
Goodwill Industries, 8, 65, 115, 144, 153
Gordon, Dr. Edward, 105
Gorgas, Dr. W. C., 15, 20
Gorodezky, Eli, 121
Gorthy, Willis, 115, 127
Graham, Dr. Evarts A., 116
Granger, Dr. Frank E., 20
Grant, Maj. Gen. David N. W., 82
Grant, Richard A., 164
Green, Rep. Edith, 144, 145
Greer, Cap. John, 86
Greer, Samuel M., 29
Greve, Bell, 112, 114, 128
Grinker, Dr. Roy M., 83

Haddan, Chester W., 121
Hamilton, Kenneth, 115
Harding, Warren G., 17, 36, 75
Harmon, John C., Jr., 144
Harrison, Frank, 38
Hartford County Rehabilitation Workship, 114
Harvey, Dr. Vern K., 113
Hawley, Maj. Gen. Paul R., 92, 93, 95
Hayes, Albert J., 116
Hayes, Charles B., 41
Health, Education and Welfare, Department of, 68, 117, 119, 130, 131, 133, 150, 151, 155, 156, 158, 168
Health Resources Advisory Committee, 112
Heber, Dr. F. Rick, 138
Held, John, 47
Helms, Edgar J., 8
Hendrix, Seid, 144
Henshel, Col. Harry D., 100
Herriot, Mayor, Lyons, 9
Heyworth, James O., 154
Hill, Sen. Lister, 137, 140, 141, 142
Hines VA hospital, 95
Hitler, Adolf, 69, 73, 91, 137
Hobby, Oveta Culp, 117
Hohenberg, Duchess of, 8
Holderman, Beatrice, 160
Hollein, Dr. Harry, 101
Hoover, Herbert Clark, 47, 48, 49, 54, 124

Hoover, Dr. Richard E., 95
Hope, Bob, 159
Hope, Walter E., 28
Hopkins, Harry, 57
Hospital for Crippled Children, Newark, 105
— Joint Diseases and Medical Center, 125
House Appropriations Committee, Subcommittee for Departments of Labor & Health, Education & Welfare, 161
— Education Committee, 34, 60
— Education and Labor Committee, 77, 78, 79, 117, 118, 119; Special Education Subcommittee 145; Special Subcommittee on Assistance & Rehabilitation of the Physically Handicapped, 118
— Ways and Means Committee, 59, 60
Howenstine, Jay, 58
Hudson, Holland, 91
Hughes Aircraft Company, 129, 130
Hughes, Charles Evans, 24
Human Resources Center, 123
Humphrey, Hubert H., 112, 143, 158
Hunt, Joseph, 156

Industrial Home for the Blind in Brooklyn, 112, 154
Institute for the Crippled & Disabled, 15, 28, 49, 54, 60, 61, 86, 87, 88, 96, 112, 115, 117, 119, 127, 128, 129, 159, 169
— of Physical Medicine & Rehabilitation (Peoria, Illinois), 162
— of Reconstructive Plastic Surgery, 129
— of Rehabilitation Medicine, NYC (Physical Medicine & Rehabilitation), 104, 106, 137
International Association of Machinists, 116
— Association of Rehabilitation Facilities, 115, 129
— Brotherhood of Boilermakers, Iron Shipbuilders, Blacksmiths, Forgers & Helpers, 163